POCKET GUIDE TO

VACCINATION AND PROPHYLAXIS

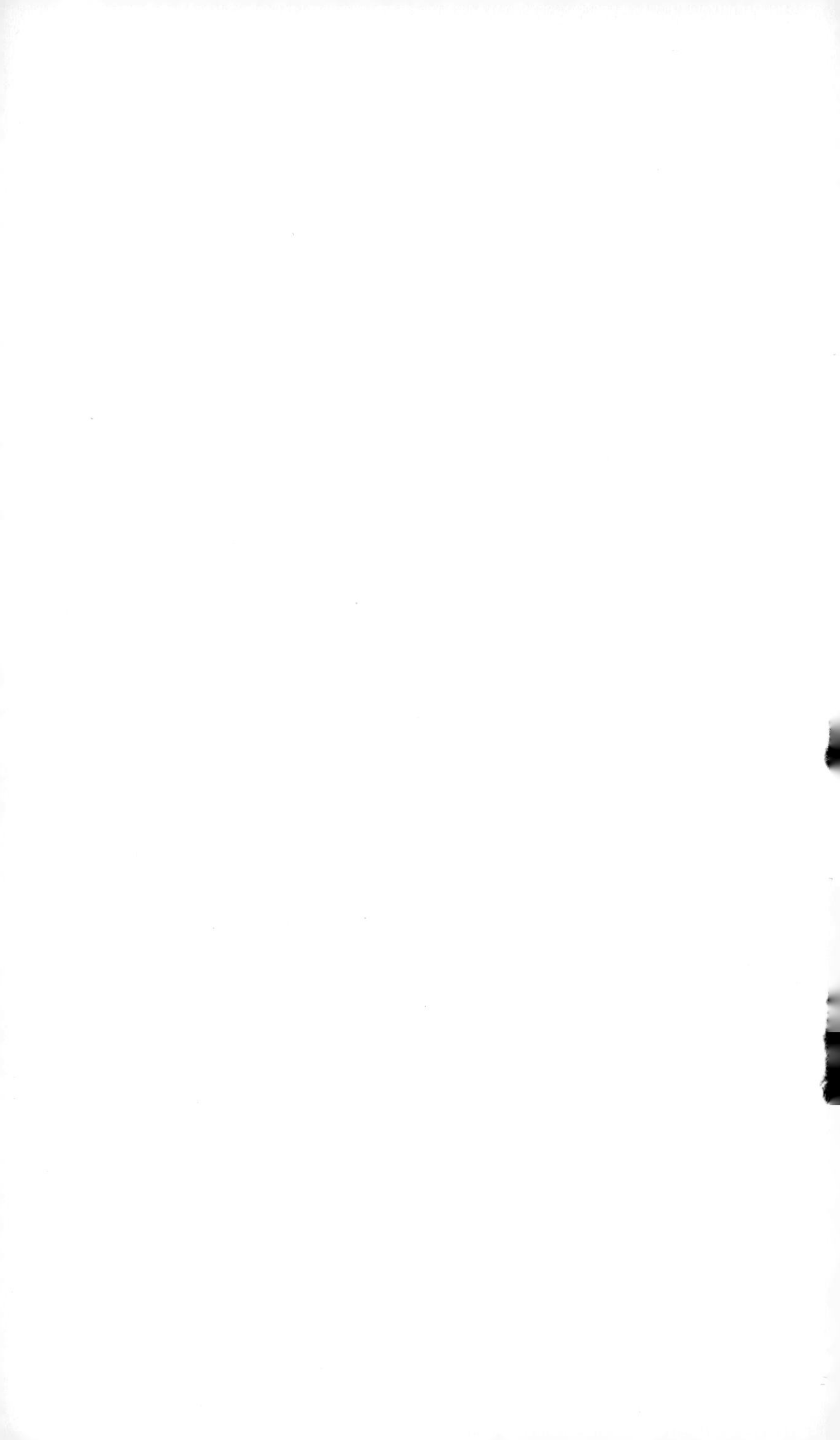

POCKET GUIDE TO VACCINATION AND PROPHYLAXIS

Hal B. Jenson, M.D.

Professor of Pediatrics and Microbiology
Chief, Pediatric Infectious Diseases
The University of Texas Health Science Center at San Antonio
San Antonio, Texas

W.B. SAUNDERS COMPANY
A Division of Harcourt Brace & Company
Philadelphia London Toronto Montreal Sydney Tokyo

W.B. SAUNDERS COMPANY

A Division of Harcourt Brace & Company

The Curtis Center
Independence Square West
Philadelphia, Pennsylvania 19106

Library of Congress Cataloging-in-Publication Data

Jenson, Hal B.
Pocket guide to vaccination and prophylaxis / Hal B. Jenson.
p. cm.
Includes bibliographical references and index.
ISBN 0-7216-7993-5
1. Vaccination—Handbooks, manuals, etc. 2. Immunization—Handbooks, manuals, etc. I. Title.
[DNLM: 1. Vaccination handbooks. 2. Immunization, Passive handbooks. 3. Vaccines—handbooks. 4. Immunoglobulins handbooks. QW 539J54p 1999]
RA638.J46 1999
615'.372—dc21
DNLM/DLC

98-38330

POCKET GUIDE TO VACCINATION AND PROPHYLAXIS ISBN 0-7216-7993-5

Printed in the United States of America

Last digit is the print number: 9 8 7 6 5 4 3 2 1

List of Abbreviations

AAFP	American Academy of Family Physicians
AAP	American Academy of Pediatrics
ACIP	Advisory Committee on Immunization Practices
ACOG	American College of Obstetricians and Gynecologists
AIDS	Acquired immunodeficiency syndrome
anti-HBs	Antibody to hepatitis B virus surface antigen
anti-HCV	Antibody to hepatitis C virus
BCG	Bacille Calmette-Guérin vaccine
CBC	Complete blood count
CDC	Centers for Disease Control and Prevention
CFU	Colony-forming units
CMV	Cytomegalovirus
CrCl	Creatinine clearance
CSF	Cerebrospinal fluid
DT	Diphtheria and tetanus toxoids, adsorbed (for pediatric use)
DTP	Diphtheria and tetanus toxoids and whole-cell pertussis vaccine, adsorbed (for pediatric use); also known as DTwP
DTaP	Diphtheria and tetanus toxoids and acellular pertussis vaccine, adsorbed (for pediatric use)
DTwP	Diphtheria and tetanus toxoids and whole-cell pertussis vaccine, adsorbed (for pediatric use); also known as DTP
EIA	Enzyme immunoassay
eIPV	Enhanced-potency inactivated poliovirus vaccine (also known as IPV)
EL.U.	Enzyme-linked immunosorbent assay (ELISA) unit
FDA	Food and Drug Administration
GBS	Group B *Streptococcus*
HA	Hemagglutination unit
HAV	Hepatitis A virus
HbOC	*Haemophilus influenzae* type b oligosaccharide conjugate
HBsAg	Hepatitis B surface antigen
HBV	Hepatitis B virus
HCV	Hepatitis C virus
HBIG	Hepatitis B immune globulin
HCW	Health-care worker

HDCV	Human diploid cell vaccine (rabies)
Hib	*Haemophilus influenzae* type b vaccine
HIV	Human immunodeficiency virus
HRIG	Human rabies immune globulin
IAP	Intrapartum antimicrobial prophylaxis
IDSA	Infectious Diseases Society of America
IG	Immune globulin for intramuscular injection (formerly known as immune serum globulin [ISG])
IPV	Inactivated poliovirus vaccine (also known as eIPV)
ISG	Immune serum globulin for intramuscular injection (now known as immune globulin [IG])
IU	International unit
IVIG	Intravenous immune globulin
Lf	Limits of flocculation
Massachusetts PHBL	Massachusetts Public Health Biologic Laboratories
Michigan BPI	Michigan Biologic Products Institute
MMR	Measles, mumps, and rubella vaccines, live
MR	Measles and rubella vaccines, live
OMP	Outer membrane protein complex of group B *Neisseria meningitidis*
OPV	Oral poliovirus vaccine, live, trivalent
ORS	Oral rehydration solution
PCP	*Pneumocystis carinii* pneumonia
PCEC	Purified chick embryo cell culture vaccine (rabies)
PCR	Polymerase chain reaction
PEP	Postexposure prophylaxis
PFU	Plaque forming units
PRP	Polysaccharide-ribitol-phosphate vaccine
RFFIT	Rapid fluorescent focus inhibition test
RIA	Radioimmunoassay
RIG	Rabies immune globulin (also known as HRIG [human rabies immune globulin])
RSV	Respiratory syncytial virus
RSV IGIV	Respiratory syncytial virus immune globulin intravenous
RVA	Rabies vaccine, adsorbed
SIDS	Sudden infant death syndrome
SMX	Sulfamethoxazole
T	Tetanus toxoid, adsorbed
TB	Tuberculosis
TCID	Tissue culture infective dose
Td	Tetanus and diphtheria toxoids, adsorbed (for children ≥7 years of age and adults)

TIG	Tetanus immune globulin
TMP	Trimethoprim
VAERS	Vaccine Adverse Events Reporting System
Var	Varicella vaccine
VZIG	Varicella-zoster immune globulin
VZV	Varicella-zoster virus
WHO	World Health Organization

NOTICE

Preface

A constant feature of clinical infectious diseases is change, and an area of great change in infectious diseases during the past several years has been with vaccines and the prevention of disease. New vaccines developed against additional infectious agents, availability of different types of vaccines against the same infectious agent, expanded indications and recommended routine use of older as well as newer vaccines, and increased international travel have combined to change the nature of what is traditionally considered as providing "routine" vaccinations. These advances have prevented many infections but have also complicated the appropriate delivery of vaccines.

The Advisory Committee on Immunization Practices of the Centers for Disease Control and Prevention, the American Academy of Pediatrics, the American College of Physicians, the American Academy of Family Physicians, the American College of Obstetricians and Gynecologists, and the American Medical Association individually and jointly have provided voluminous written specific recommendations and guidelines for appropriate use of vaccines, immune globulin products, and antimicrobial agents for prevention of infectious diseases. The Infectious Diseases Society of America has also commissioned a series of practice guidelines related to vaccine use and prophylaxis of infection. The statements from these national bodies have been strong and have become established as standards of care.

This pocket guide provides a compact compendium of the recommended uses of vaccines, immune globulin products, antimicrobial agents, and other measures for prevention of disease in children, adolescents, and adults based on these policies. This guide is intended to provide quick access to these standards by organizing this information in comprehensive but simplified tables. Additional detailed information is available from the sources listed for each table and from the references listed at the end of the *Pocket Guide,* as well as from standard texts of medicine, pediatrics, and infectious diseases.

The occasional differences in recommendations between different professional organizations and the few instances of standard practice that have not been formally stated by these national bodies are indicated. Updated information to this pocket guide is available on the Internet at www.vaccine.uthsca.edu. I hope that this pocket guide serves as a practical resource in the office, clinic, and hospital. I welcome suggestions for improving the usability of this guide.

Hal B. Jenson, M.D.

Chief, Division of Pediatric Infectious Diseases
University of Texas Health Science Center
San Antonio, TX 78284-7811
jenson@uthsca.edu

Contents

VACCINATIONS

Vaccinations

Childhood Immunizations

RECOMMENDED CHILDHOOD IMMUNIZATION SCHEDULE
UNITED STATES, JANUARY–DECEMBER 1998

Age ▶ Vaccine[1] ▼	Birth	1 mo	2 mo	4 mo	6 mo	12 mo	15 mo	18 mo	4–6 yr	11–12 yr	14–16 yr
Hepatitis B[2,3]	Hep B-1										
		Hep B-2			Hep B-3					Hep B[3]	
Diphtheria, tetanus, pertussis[4]			DTaP or DTP	DTaP or DTP	DTaP or DTP		DTaP or DTP[4]		DTaP or DTP	Td	
Haemophilus influenzae type b[5]			Hib	Hib	Hib	Hib					
Polio[6]			Polio[6]	Polio	Polio[6]				Polio		
Rotavirus[7]			RV	RV	RV						
Measles, mumps, rubella[8]						MMR			MMR	MMR[8]	
Varicella[9]						Var				Var[9]	

See legend on next page

Approved by the Advisory Committee on Immunization Practices (ACIP), the American Academy of Pediatrics (AAP), and the American Academy of Family Physicians (AAFP).

Adapted from Centers for Disease Control and Prevention: Recommended childhood immunization schedule—United States, 1998. *MMWR Morb Mortal Wkly Rep* 1998;47:10–11.

[1]This schedule indicates the recommended age for routine administration of currently licensed childhood vaccines; vaccines are listed under the ages for which they are routinely recommended. Bars indicate the range of acceptable ages for immunization. Catch-up immunization should be done during any visit when feasible. Shaded ovals indicate vaccines to be assessed and given if necessary during the early adolescent visit. Combination vaccines (page 74) may be used whenever any components of the combination are indicated and its other components are not contraindicated. Providers should consult the manufacturers' package inserts for detailed recommendations.

[2]***Infants born to HBsAg-negative mothers*** should receive 5 μg of Merck vaccine (Recombivax HB) or 10 μg of SmithKline Beecham vaccine (Engerix-B). The second dose should be administered at least 1 month after the first dose. The third dose should be administered at least 2 months after the second dose but not before the child is 6 months of age.

Infants born to HBsAg-positive mothers should receive 0.5 mL hepatitis B immune globulin (HBIG) within 12 hours of birth and either 5 μg of Merck vaccine (Recombivax HB) or 10 μg of SmithKline Beecham vaccine (Engerix-B) at a separate site. The second dose is recommended at 1–2 months of age and the third dose at 6 months of age (page 205).

Infants born to mothers whose HBsAg status is unknown should receive either 5 μg of Merck vaccine (Recombivax HB) or 10 μg of SmithKline Beecham vaccine (Engerix-B) within 12 hours of birth. The second dose of vaccine is recommended at 1–2 months of age and the third dose at 6 months of age. Blood should be drawn at the time of delivery to determine the mother's HBsAg status; if it is positive, the infant should receive HBIG as soon as possible (no later than 1 week of age). The dosage and timing of subsequent vaccine doses should be based on the mother's HBsAg status (page 59).

Legend continued on following page

[3]Children and adolescents who have not been vaccinated against hepatitis B in infancy may begin the series during any visit. Those who have not previously received 3 doses of hepatitis B vaccine should initiate or complete the series during the routine visit to a health-care provider at 11–12 years of age, and unvaccinated older adolescents should be vaccinated whenever possible. The second dose should be administered at least 1 month after the first dose, and the third dose should be administered at least 4 months after the first dose and at least 2 months after the second dose.

[4]DTaP (diphtheria and tetanus toxoids and acellular pertussis vaccine) is the preferred vaccine for all doses in the vaccination series, including completion of the series in children who have received 1 or more doses of DTP (diphtheria and tetanus toxoids and whole-cell pertussis vaccine). Whole-cell DTP is an acceptable alternative to DTaP. The fourth dose (DTaP or DTP) may be administered as early as 12 months of age if 6 months have elapsed since the third dose and if the child is unlikely to return at 15–18 months of age. Td (tetanus and diphtheria toxoids, for adult use) is recommended at 11–12 years of age if at least 5 years have elapsed since the last dose of DTP, DTaP, or DT (tetanus and diphtheria toxoids, for pediatric use). Subsequent routine Td (tetanus and diphtheria toxoids, for adult use) boosters are recommended every 10 years.

[5]Three *Haemophilus influenzae* type b (Hib) conjugate vaccines are licensed for infant use. If PRP-OMP (PedvaxHIB [Merck]) is administered at 2 and 4 months of age, a dose at 6 months of age is not required.

[6]Two poliovirus vaccines are currently licensed in the United States: inactivated poliovirus vaccine (IPV) and oral poliovirus vaccine (OPV). The following schedules are all acceptable to the ACIP, the AAP, and the AAFP. Parents and providers may choose among these options (page 67):

1. Two doses of IPV followed by two doses of OPV
2. Four doses of IPV
3. Four doses of OPV

The ACIP recommends 2 doses of IPV at 2 and 4 months of age followed by 2 doses of OPV at 12–18 months and 4–6 years of age. The AAP and AAFP give no preference for any of the three acceptable schedules and recommend that, for children who received IPV at ages 2 and 4 months, the third dose of polio vaccine (either IPV or OPV) be administered at 6–18 months of age. IPV is the only poliovirus vaccine recommended for immunocompromised persons and their household contacts.

[7]The ACIP made a preliminary recommendation in February 1998 for routine use of the rotavirus vaccine. Rotavirus vaccine received FDA approval on August 31, 1998. Final ACIP/CDC, AAP, and AAFP recommendations are pending as of September 1, 1998. For updated information, see www.vaccine.uthscsa.edu.

[8]The second dose of MMR (measles, mumps, and rubella vaccine) is recommended routinely at 4–6 years of age but may be administered during any visit if at least 1 month has elapsed since receipt of the first dose and both doses are administered beginning at or after 12 months of age. Children who have not previously received the second dose should complete the schedule no later than the routine visit to a health-care provider at 11–12 years of age.

[9]Susceptible children may receive Var (varicella vaccine) at any visit after the first birthday, and those who lack a reliable history of chickenpox should be immunized during the routine visit to a health-care provider at 11–12 years of age. Susceptible children ≥13 years of age should receive 2 doses at least 1 month apart.

RECOMMENDED IMMUNIZATION SCHEDULE FOR CHILDREN BEHIND IN IMMUNIZATION

Recommended Accelerated Immunization Schedule for Infants and Children <7 Years of Age Who Start the Series Late or Who Are More Than 1 Month Behind in the Immunization Schedule (i.e., Children for Whom Compliance with Scheduled Return Visits Cannot Be Assured)[1]

Timing	Vaccine(s)
First visit (≥4 months of age)	DTaP (or DTP),[2] OPV,[3] Hib,[2,4] hepatitis B, MMR (as soon as child is 12–15 months old)
Second visit (1 month after the first visit)	DTaP (or DTP),[2] hepatitis B, varicella
Third visit (1 month after the second visit)	DTaP (or DTP),[2] OPV, Hib[2,4]
Fourth visit (6 weeks after the third visit)	OPV
Fifth visit (≥6 months after the third visit)	DTaP or DTP,[2] Hib,[2,4] hepatitis B
Additional visits	
4–6 years of age	DTaP (or DTP), OPV, MMR
11–16 years of age and repeated every 10 years throughout life	Td

Adapted from Centers for Disease Control and Prevention. General recommendations on immunization. Recommendations of the Advisory Committee on Immunization Practices (ACIP). *MMWR Morb Mortal Wkly Rep* 1994;43 (RR-1):10.

[1]See individual ACIP recommendations for detailed information on specific vaccines.

[2]Two DTP and Hib combination vaccines (page 74) are available: Tetramune (HbOC/DTwP) for all doses; and TriHIBit, which combines PRP-T (ActHIB, OmniHIB), reconstituted with DTaP vaccine produced by Connaught (Tripedia) for the booster (fourth dose) of DTP in children ≥15 months of age. DTP and DTaP should not be used for children ≥7 years of age.

[3]For infants and children starting vaccination late (i.e., after 6 months of age), IPV is also acceptable, although OPV is preferred to complete an accelerated schedule with a minimum number of injections.

[4]The recommended schedule varies by vaccine manufacturer (page 53). For information specific to the vaccine being used, consult the package insert and ACIP recommendations. Children beginning the Hib vaccine series at age 2–6 months should receive a primary series of three doses of HbOC (HibTITER [Lederle]), PRP-T (ActHIB, OmniHIB [Pasteur-Mérieux; SmithKline Beecham; Connaught]), or a licensed DTP-Hib combination vaccine (page 74); or 2 doses of PRP-OMP (PedvaxHIB [Merck]). An additional booster dose of any licensed Hib conjugate vaccine should be administered at 12–15 months of age and at least 2 months after the previous dose. Children beginning the Hib vaccine series at 7–11 months of age should receive a primary series of two doses of an HbOC-, PRP-T–, or PRP-OMP–containing vaccine. An additional booster dose of any licensed Hib conjugate vaccine should be administered at 12–18 months of age and at least 2 months after the previous dose. Children beginning licensed Hib conjugate vaccine should be given the second dose 2 months after the previous dose. Children beginning the Hib vaccine series at 15–59 months of age should receive 1 dose of any licensed Hib vaccine. Hib vaccine should not be administered after the fifth birthday except for special circumstances as noted in the specific ACIP recommendations for the use of Hib vaccine.

Recommended Immunization Schedule for Persons ≥7 Years of Age Who Were Not Vaccinated at the Recommended Time in Early Infancy[1]

Timing	Vaccine(s)
First visit	Td,[2] OPV,[3] MMR,[4] hepatitis B[5]
Second visit (6–8 weeks after the first visit)	Td, OPV, MMR,[4,6] hepatitis B[5], varicella[7]
Third visit (6 months after the second visit)	Td, OPV, hepatitis B[5]
11–16 years of age and repeated every 10 years throughout life	Td

Adapted from Centers for Disease Control and Prevention. General recommendations on immunization. Recommendations of the Advisory Committee on Immunization Practices (ACIP). *MMWR Morb Mortal Wkly Rep* 1994;43 (RR-1):11.

[1]See individual ACIP recommendations for detailed information on specific vaccines.

[2]The DTP and DTaP doses administered to children < 7 years of age who remain incompletely vaccinated at 7 years of age or older should be counted as prior vaccination with tetanus and diphtheria toxoids (e.g., a child who previously received 2 doses of DTP needs only 1 dose of Td to complete a primary series for tetanus and diphtheria).

[3]For children starting vaccination late, IPV is also acceptable, although OPV is preferred to complete an accelerated schedule with the minimum number of injections. Primary poliovirus vaccination is not routinely recommended for persons ≥18 years of age. When polio vaccine is administered to previously unvaccinated persons ≥18 years of age, inactivated poliovirus vaccine (IPV) is preferred (page 63).

[4]Persons born before 1957 can generally be considered immune to measles and mumps and need not be vaccinated. Rubella (or MMR) vaccine is recommended for all rubella-susceptible nonpregnant women of childbearing age.

[5]Hepatitis B vaccine is indicated for all adolescents and for selected high-risk groups (page 56).

[6]Children with no documentation of live measles vaccination after the first birthday should receive 2 doses of live measles–containing vaccine (preferably MMR to ensure immunity to mumps and rubella) not less than 1 month apart. In addition, the following persons born in 1957 or later should have documentation of measles immunity (i.e., 2 doses of measles-containing vaccine [at least one of which is MMR], physician-diagnosed measles, or laboratory evidence of measles immunity): (a) those entering post–high school education; (b) those beginning employment in health-care settings who will have direct patient contact; and (c) travelers to areas with endemic measles.

[7]Unvaccinated children who lack a reliable history of chickenpox should be vaccinated with varicella vaccine before their 13th birthday.

Immunization of Adolescents

Recommended Routine Vaccinations for Adolescents (at 11–12 Years of Age)

Universally indicated

Hepatitis B vaccine (page 56)

- Adolescents 11–12 years of age who have not been vaccinated previously and unvaccinated adolescents >12 years of age at increased risk for hepatitis B infection
- Primary schedule: Recombivax HB (5 μg/0.5 mL) or Engerix-B (20 μg/1 mL): 3 doses intramuscularly at 0, 1–2, and 4–6 months

Measles, mumps, and rubella vaccine (MMR) (page 60)

- Adolescents not vaccinated previously with 2 doses of measles vaccine at ≥12 months of age
- Primary schedule: MMR, 0.5 mL subcutaneously, 2 doses separated by at least 1 month

Tetanus and diphtheria toxoids (Td) (page 47)

- Adolescents not vaccinated within the previous 5 years
- Booster schedule: tetanus and diphtheria toxoids, adsorbed (for adult use), 0.5 mL intramuscularly every 10 years throughout life

Varicella vaccine (page 71)

- Adolescents not vaccinated previously and who have no reliable history of chickenpox
- Primary schedule: Varivax, 0.5 mL subcutaneously:
  - Age <13 years: 1 dose
  - Age ≥13 years: 2 doses separated by 4–8 weeks

Adapted from Centers for Disease Control and Prevention. Immunization of adolescents. Recommendations of the Advisory Committee on Immunization Practices, the American Academy of Pediatrics, the American Academy of Family Practice, and the American Medical Association. *MMWR Morb Mortal Wkly Rep* 1996;45 (RR-13):5.

Indicated for adolescents in high-risk groups

Hepatitis A vaccine (page 76)

- Adolescents who are at increased risk of hepatitis A infection or its complications (page 76)
- Primary schedule:
  - Havrix: 2 doses of 720 EL.U./0.5 mL intramuscularly, separated by 6–12 months[1]
  - Vaqta: 2 doses of 25 U/0.5 mL intramuscularly, separated by 6–18 months[2]

Influenza vaccine (page 79)

- Adolescents who are at increased risk for complications of influenza (page 79) or who have contact with persons at increased risk for complications of influenza
- Primary schedule: influenza vaccine, 0.5 mL intramuscularly, annually administered between October 1 and mid-November (any time from September to the end of the influenza season, as long as cases are still occurring and if the person is not previously immunized, is appropriate)

Pneumococcus vaccine (page 83)

- Adolescents who are at increased risk for pneumococcal disease or its complications (page 83)
- Primary schedule: pneumococcus vaccine, 0.5 mL intramuscularly or subcutaneously (with revaccination as indicated on page 85)

EL.U. = enzyme-linked immunosorbent assay (ELISA) unit.

[1]Adults >18 years of age should receive Havrix, 1440 EL.U./1 mL, 2 doses at 0 and 6–12 months.

[2]Adults ≥18 years of age should receive Vaqta, 50 U/1 mL, 2 doses at 0 and 6 months.

Immunization of Adults

Overview of Recommended Routine Vaccinations for Adults

	Vaccine/Toxoid				
Age-group (years)	**Td[1] (every 10 years)**	**Measles, Mumps, and Rubella**	**Varicella**	**Influenza (annually)**	**Pneumococcus**
18–24	Yes	Yes[2]	If susceptible[3]	If in a high-risk group	If in a high-risk group
25–64	Yes	Yes, for persons born during or after 1957 or in a high-risk group[2]	If susceptible[3]	If in a high-risk group	If in a high-risk group
≥65	Yes	Not required for most adults born before 1957	If susceptible[3]	Yes	Yes

Adapted from Centers for Disease Control. Update on adult immunization. Recommendations of the Immunization Practices Advisory Committee (ACIP). *MMWR Morb Mortal Wkly Rep* 1991;40 (RR-12):56.

[1]Td = Tetanus and diphtheria toxoids, adsorbed (for adult use), which is a combined preparation containing <2 flocculation units of diphtheria toxoid.

[2]One dose of MMR for all persons born in 1957 or later, two doses of live measles vaccine (as MMR) for college or university students, health-care workers (page 24), or international travelers. Birth before 1957 is not acceptable evidence for immunity to rubella for women who can become pregnant. Rubella vaccination with one dose of live rubella vaccine (as MMR) is indicated for all females who can become pregnant who lack appropriate vaccination or laboratory evidence of rubella immunity.

[3]Adults of any age without a reliable history of varicella disease or vaccination, or who have serologic evidence of susceptibility.

Recommended Routine Vaccinations for Adults

Universally indicated

Tetanus and diphtheria toxoids (Td) (page 47)

- Adults not vaccinated within the previous 10 years
- Booster schedule: tetanus and diphtheria toxoids, adsorbed (for adult use), 0.5 mL intramuscularly every 10 years throughout life

Measles, mumps, and rubella vaccine (MMR) (page 60)

- Adults born during or after 1957 or later without documentation of (a) physician-diagnosed measles or mumps disease; or (b) laboratory evidence of measles, mumps, or rubella immunity (persons who have an "indeterminate" level of immunity upon testing should be considered nonimmune); or (c) appropriate vaccination against measles, mumps, and rubella (i.e., administration on or after the first birthday of two doses of live measles vaccine separated by ≥28 days, at least one dose of live mumps vaccine, and at least one dose of live rubella vaccine)
- Primary schedule: MMR, 0.5 mL subcutaneously, 1 dose for all persons born in 1957 or later; for college or university students, health-care workers (page 24), or international travelers, 2 doses at least 1 month apart

Varicella vaccine (page 71)

- Adults of any age without a reliable history of varicella disease or vaccination or who have serologic evidence of susceptibility
- Primary schedule: Varivax, 0.5 mL subcutaneously, for a total of 2 doses separated by 4–8 weeks

Universally indicated for adults ≥65 years of age

Influenza vaccine (page 79)

- Adults who are at increased risk for complications of influenza (page 79) or who have contact with persons at increased risk for complications of influenza

---

Adapted from Centers for Disease Control. Update on adult immunization. Recommendations of the Immunization Practices Advisory Committee (ACIP). *MMWR Morb Mortal Wkly Rep* 1991;40 (RR-12):1–94.

- Primary schedule: influenza vaccine, 0.5 mL intramuscularly annually administered between October 1 and mid-November (any time from September to the end of the influenza season, as long as cases are still occurring and if the person is not previously immunized, is appropriate)

Pneumococcus vaccine (page 83)

- Adults who are at increased risk for pneumococcal disease or its complications (page 83)
- Primary schedule: pneumococcus vaccine, 0.5 mL intramuscularly or subcutaneously (with revaccination as indicated on page 85)

Indicated for adults in high-risk groups

Hepatitis A vaccine (page 76)

- Adults who are at increased risk of hepatitis A infection or its complications (page 76)
- Primary schedule:
  - Havrix: 2 doses of 1440 EL.U./1 mL intramuscularly, separated by 6–12 months[1]
  - Vaqta: 2 doses of 50 U/1 mL intramuscularly, separated by 6 months[2]

Hepatitis B vaccine (page 56)

- Adults in high-risk groups who are at increased risk of hepatitis B infection or its complications (page 56)
- Primary schedule: Recombivax HB (10 μg/1 mL) or Engerix-B (20 μg/1 mL): 3 doses intramuscularly at 0, 1–2, 4–6 months

Poliovirus vaccine (page 63)

- Unimmunized or partially immunized adults in high-risk groups or who have contact with persons at increased risk (page 63) (adults ≥18 years of age residing in the United States who never received or completed a primary series of polio vaccine do not need to be vaccinated unless otherwise indicated)

---

[1]Adolescents ≤18 years of age should receive Havrix, 720 EL.U./0.5 mL, 2 doses at 0 and 6–12 months.

[2]Adolescents <18 years of age should receive Vaqta, 25 U/0.5 mL, 2 doses at 0 and 6 months.

Vaccinations Recommended for Adults for Special Circumstances

Occupations	
Hospital, laboratory, and other health-care personnel (page 24)	Hepatitis B Influenza Measles Mumps Rubella Polio Varicella (if not already immune)
Public-safety personnel	Hepatitis B Influenza
Staff of institutions for developmentally disabled people	Hepatitis B
Veterinarians and animal handlers	Plague Rabies
Selected field workers (those who come into contact with possibly infected animals)	Plague Rabies
Selected occupations (those who work with imported animal hides, furs, wool, animal hair, and bristles)	Anthrax
Life-styles	
Homosexual males	Hepatitis B
Injecting drug users	Hepatitis B
Heterosexual persons with multiple sexual partners or recently acquired sexually transmitted disease	Hepatitis B
Inmates of long-term correctional facilities	Hepatitis B
Residents of institutions for developmentally disabled people	Hepatitis B
Household contacts of HBV (HBsAg) carriers	Hepatitis B
Homeless persons	Tetanus/diphtheria Measles Mumps Rubella Influenza Pneumococcus
Foreign students, immigrants, and refugees	Diphtheria Tetanus Measles Mumps Rubella Hepatitis B

Health Conditions	
Pregnant women	Tetanus/diphtheria
Hemodialysis or organ transplant recipients	Hepatitis B Influenza Pneumococcus
Immunocompromised persons (page 34)	Influenza Pneumococcus *Haemophilus influenzae* type b
Persons with splenic dysfunction or anatomical asplenia	Pneumococcus Influenza Meningococcus *Haemophilus influenzae* type b
Persons with deficiencies of factor VIII or IX	Hepatitis B
Persons with chronic alcoholism	Hepatitis B
Persons with diabetes or other high-risk diseases	Influenza Pneumococcus

Adapted from Centers for Disease Control. Update on adult immunization. Recommendations of the Immunization Practices Advisory Committee (ACIP). *MMWR Morb Mortal Wkly Rep* 1991;40 (RR-12):57–58.

Use of Vaccines and Immune Globulins during Pregnancy

Immunobiological	Risk from Disease to Pregnant Female	Risk from Disease to Fetus or Neonate	Risk from Immunizing Agent to Fetus	Indications for Immunization during Pregnancy	Comments
Live-Virus Vaccines					
Japanese encephalitis (page 96)	Significant morbidity and mortality (not altered by pregnancy)	Possible intrauterine infection and fetal death	Unknown	Contraindicated except if travel to an area where the risk of Japanese encephalitis is high	Postponement of travel preferable to vaccination, if possible
Measles (page 60)	Significant morbidity, low mortality (not altered by pregnancy)	Significant increase in abortion rate; may cause malformation	None confirmed	Contraindicated	Vaccination of susceptible women should be part of postpartum care
Mumps (page 60)	Low morbidity and mortality (not altered by pregnancy)	Probable increased rate of abortion in first trimester; questionable association of fibroelastosis in neonates	None confirmed	Contraindicated	

Rubella (page 60)	Low morbidity and mortality (not altered by pregnancy)	High rate of abortion and congenital rubella syndrome	None confirmed	Contraindicated	Teratogenicity of vaccine is theoretical, not confirmed to date; vaccination of susceptible women should be part of postpartum care
Yellow fever (page 100)	Significant morbidity and mortality (not altered by pregnancy)	Unknown	Unknown	Contraindicated except if exposure to yellow fever virus is unavoidable	Postponement of travel preferable to vaccination, if possible
Varicella (page 71)	Significant morbidity and mortality (may be exacerbated by pregnancy)	Significant risk with onset of maternal rash of chickenpox within 5 days before delivery to within 48 hours after delivery	None confirmed	Contraindicated	

Table continued on following page

Immunobiological	Risk from Disease to Pregnant Female	Risk from Disease to Fetus or Neonate	Risk from Immunizing Agent to Fetus	Indications for Immunization during Pregnancy	Comments
Toxoids					
Tetanus/diphtheria (page 47)	Severe morbidity; tetanus mortality, 60%; diphtheria mortality, 10% (both of which are not altered by pregnancy)	Neonatal tetanus mortality, 60%	None confirmed	Lack of primary series or no booster within past 10 years	Updating of immune status should be part of antepartum care; unvaccinated women should be vaccinated, preferably after first trimester
Inactivated-Virus and Live-Virus Vaccines					
Poliomyelitis (page 63)	No increased incidence in pregnancy but may be more severe if it does occur	Anoxic fetal damage reported; 50% mortality in neonatal disease	None confirmed	Not routinely recommended for adults in United States, except persons at increased risk of exposure	OPV indicated for susceptible pregnant women traveling in endemic areas or in other high-risk situations; no data on safety of eIPV in pregnancy

Inactivated-Virus Vaccines					
Hepatitis B (page 56)	Possible increased severity during third trimester	Possible increase in abortion rate and prematurity; perinatal transmission may occur if mother is a chronic carrier or is acutely infected; newborns are at risk of fulminant hepatitis or of becoming chronic carrier	None reported	Indications for prophylaxis not altered by pregnancy	Infants born to HBsAg-positive mothers should receive HBIG and hepatitis B vaccine as soon as possible after birth (page 205)
Influenza (page 79)	Increased complications during second and third trimesters	Possible increased abortion rate; no malformation confirmed	None confirmed	Women who will be in the second or third trimester (≥14 weeks' gestation) of pregnancy during the influenza season (December through March)	Pregnant women who have medical conditions that increase their risk for complications from influenza should be vaccinated before the influenza season regardless of the stage of pregnancy

Table continued on following page

Immunobiological	Risk from Disease to Pregnant Female	Risk from Disease to Fetus or Neonate	Risk from Immunizing Agent to Fetus	Indications for Immunization during Pregnancy	Comments
Rabies (page 86)	Near 100% fatality (not altered by pregnancy)	Determined by maternal disease	Unknown	Indications for prophylaxis not altered by pregnancy; each case considered individually	
Inactivated-Bacteria Vaccines					
Cholera (page 94)	Significant morbidity and mortality; more severe during third trimester	Increased risk of fetal death during maternal illness in third trimester	Unknown	Only to meet international travel requirements	Vaccine of low efficacy
Meningococcus (page 82)	No increased risk during pregnancy; no increase in severity of disease	Unknown	No data available on use during pregnancy	Indications not altered by pregnancy; vaccination recommended only in unusual outbreak situations	
Plague (page 98)	Significant morbidity and mortality (not altered by pregnancy)	Determined by maternal disease	None reported	Very selective vaccination of exposed persons	

Pneumococcus (page 83)	No increased risk during pregnancy; no increase in severity of disease	Unknown	No data available on use during pregnancy	Indications not altered by pregnancy; vaccine used only for persons at high risk	
Typhoid (page 89)	Significant morbidity and mortality (not altered by pregnancy)	Unknown	None confirmed	Not recommended routinely except for close, continued exposure or travel to areas where disease is endemic	
Immune Globulins					
Hepatitis A (IG, page 147)	Possible increased severity during third trimester	Possible increase in abortion rate and prematurity; possible transmission to neonate at delivery if mother is incubating the virus or is acutely ill at that time	None reported	Postexposure prophylaxis (page 164)	IG should be given as soon as possible and within 2 weeks of exposure; infants who are incubating the virus or are acutely ill at delivery should receive 1 dose of 0.5 mL as soon as possible after birth

Table continued on following page

Immunobiological	Risk from Disease to Pregnant Female	Risk from Disease to Fetus or Neonate	Risk from Immunizing Agent to Fetus	Indications for Immunization during Pregnancy	Comments
Hepatitis B (HBIG, page 152)	Possible increased severity during third trimester	Possible increase in abortion rate and prematurity; perinatal transmission may occur if mother is a chronic carrier or is acutely infected; newborns are at risk of fulminant hepatitis or chronic carriage	None reported	Postexposure prophylaxis (page 166)	Infants born to HBsAg-positive mothers should receive HBIG and hepatitis B vaccine as soon as possible after birth (page 205)
Measles (IG, page 147)	Significant morbidity, low mortality (not altered by pregnancy)	Significant increase in abortion rate; may cause malformations	None reported	Postexposure prophylaxis (page 180)	Unclear if IG prevents abortion; must be given within 6 days of exposure
Rabies (RIG, page 153)	Near 100% fatality (not altered by pregnancy)	Determined by maternal disease	None reported	Postexposure prophylaxis (page 183)	Used with rabies killed-virus vaccine
Tetanus (TIG, page 156)	Severe morbidity; mortality, 60%	Neonatal tetanus mortality, 60%	None reported	Postexposure prophylaxis (page 186)	Used with tetanus toxoid

Varicella (VZIG, page 157)	Possible increase in severe varicella pneumonia	Can cause neonatal varicella with increased mortality in neonatal period; very rarely causes congenital defects	None reported	Not routinely indicated in healthy pregnant women exposed to varicella; approximately 90%–95% of adults are immune to varicella (page 193)	Primarily indicated for newborns of mothers who had varicella within 5 days before delivery or 48 hours after delivery (page 210)

Adapted from Centers for Disease Control and Prevention. Update on adult immunization. Recommendations of the Immunization Practices Advisory Committee (ACIP). *MMWR Morb Mortal Wkly Rep* 1991;40 (RR-12):82–88.

Immunizations and Immunoprophylaxis of Health-Care Workers (HCWs)[1]

Diseases for which immunization is strongly recommended because of special risks to health-care workers

Hepatitis B

- HCWs at risk for exposure to blood or body fluids[2]
- For public-safety workers whose exposure to blood is infrequent, timely postexposure prophylaxis should be considered rather than routine preexposure vaccination

Influenza[3]

- Annual immunization in the fall of each year for:
  - HCWs who have contact with patients at risk for influenza or its complications
  - HCWs who work in chronic-care facilities or nursing homes
  - HCWs who are ≥65 years of age or have high-risk medical conditions (page 79)

Measles[4]

- HCWs born during or after 1957 who:
  - Do not have documentation of receiving 2 doses of live vaccine on or after the first birthday

---

Adapted from Centers for Disease Control and Prevention. Immunization of health-care workers. Recommendations of the Advisory Committee on Immunization Practices (ACIP) and the Hospital Infection Control Practices Advisory Committee (HICPAC). *MMWR Morb Mortal Wkly Rep* 1997;46 (RR-18):1–42.

[1]HCWs in private practice offices, nursing homes, schools, and laboratories and first responders.

[2]Prevaccination serological screening for prior infection is not indicated for persons being vaccinated because of occupational risk. Postvaccination testing for antibody to hepatitis B surface antigen (anti-HBs) response is indicated for HCWs who have blood or patient contact and are at ongoing risk for injuries with sharp instruments or needle sticks (e.g., physicians, nurses, dentists, phlebotomists, medical technicians, and students of these professions). Knowledge of antibody response aids in determining appropriate postexposure prophylaxis.

[3]Reduces staff illness and absenteeism during the influenza season and also reduces nosocomial infections.

[4]All HCWs (i.e., medical or nonmedical, paid or volunteer, full-time or part-time, student or nonstudent, with or without patient-care responsibilities) who work in facilities that provide health care to patients (i.e., inpatient or outpatient, public or private) should be immune to measles, rubella, and varicella. Facilities that provide care exclusively for elderly patients who are at minimal risk for measles and rubella and complications of these diseases are a possible exception.

  - Do not have a history of physician-diagnosed measles
  - Do not have serological evidence of measles immunity
  - Were vaccinated during 1963–1967 with a killed measles vaccine alone, with a killed measles vaccine followed by a live vaccine, or with a vaccine of unknown type
- Although birth before 1957 is generally considered evidence of measles immunity in the general population, vaccination should be considered for all HCWs who lack proof of immunity, including those born before 1957
- Two doses of measles live-virus vaccine or MMR vaccine, 1 month apart; MMR is the vaccination of choice if the recipient is likely to be susceptible to rubella or mumps as well as to measles

Mumps

- HCWs believed to be susceptible to mumps; individuals born before 1957 can be considered immune
- One dose of mumps live-virus vaccine; MMR is the vaccine of choice if the recipient is likely to be susceptible to measles or rubella as well as to mumps

Rubella[4]

- HCWs (male and female) who:
  - Do not have documentation of receiving 1 dose of live vaccine on or after the first birthday
  - Do not have serologic evidence of rubella immunity
  - Were vaccinated during 1963–1967 with a killed measles vaccine alone, with a killed measles vaccine followed by a live vaccine, or with a vaccine of unknown type
- Adults born before 1957, **except women who can become pregnant**, can be considered immune
- One dose of rubella live-virus vaccine or MMR vaccine; MMR is the vaccination of choice if the recipient is likely to be susceptible to measles or mumps as well as to rubella

Varicella[4]

- HCWs who do not have either a reliable history of varicella or serological evidence of varicella immunity[5]

---

[5]Because 71%–93% of persons without a history of varicella are immune, serological testing before vaccination is likely to be cost effective.

Bacille Calmette-Guérin (BCG)

- HCWs in areas where multidrug tuberculosis is prevalent, where a strong likelihood of exposure exists, and where comprehensive infection control precautions have been implemented but have failed to prevent tuberculosis transmission to HCWs
- Vaccination with BCG should not be routinely recommended or required for employment in specific work areas

Diseases for which immunoprophylaxis is or may be indicated in certain circumstances

Hepatitis A

- Routine preexposure prophylaxis (vaccination) of all HCWs is not recommended
- Persons who work with hepatitis A–infected primates or hepatitis A virus in a research laboratory setting
- In documented outbreaks of hepatitis A infection, IG postexposure prophylaxis (page 164) is recommended for HCWs who are exposed to feces of infected patients and who do not use proper precautions

Meningococcus

- Routine preexposure prophylaxis (vaccination) of all HCWs is not recommended
- Postexposure prophylaxis (page 178) for HCWs who have intensive contact with oropharyngeal secretions of infected patients and who do not use proper precautions
- Control of serogroup C meningococcal outbreaks with unusual clustering of serogroup C meningococcal disease

Pertussis

- Vaccination of adults with pertussis vaccines is not recommended because of adverse events of the whole-cell pertussis vaccines in persons ≥7 years of age
- Booster doses of acellular pertussis vaccines are currently licensed for children 6 weeks to 6 years of age (use in HCWs may be recommended in the future if reformulated vaccine is licensed for use in adults)

Poliovirus

- A once-per-lifetime booster of IPV (OPV may also be used for persons who have received OPV or IPV previously) for HCWs at future risk of exposure to poliomyelitis (e.g., international travel)

- HCWs directly providing care to patients who may be excreting poliovirus
- Laboratory workers who handle specimens that may contain polioviruses

Typhoid

- Routine preexposure prophylaxis (vaccination) of all HCWs is not recommended
- Workers in microbiology laboratories who frequently work with *Salmonella typhi* (Vaccination is not an alterative to the use of proper procedures when handling specimens and cultures in the laboratory.)

Vaccinia

- Routine preexposure prophylaxis (vaccination) of all HCWs is not recommended
- Laboratory workers (primarily researchers) who directly handle cultures of vaccinia, recombinant vaccinia viruses, or orthopoxviruses
- May be considered for other HCWs whose contact with orthopoxviruses is limited to contaminated dressings or other infectious materials

Diseases for which protection is recommended for all adults

Diphtheria and tetanus

- Vaccination and boosters should be provided as indicated for all adults (page 47)

Pneumococcus vaccine

- Vaccination and boosters should be provided as indicated for all adults (page 83)

Other

Hepatitis C

- No vaccine is currently available, and available immune globulin products do not protect against hepatitis C infection (all blood is tested for anti–hepatitis C antibody and excluded if positive)
- HCWs with exposure to hepatitis C–positive blood should have appropriate follow-up (page 169)
- HCWs with serological evidence of hepatitis C infection should not have restrictions but should follow strict aseptic techniques and standard precautions, including hand washing, use of protective barriers, and care in the use and disposal of needles and other sharp instruments

Immunization of Health-Care Workers with Special Conditions

Vaccine	Pregnancy	HIV Infection	Severe Immuno-suppression[1]	Asplenia	Renal Failure	Diabetes	Alcoholism and Alcoholic Cirrhosis
BCG	**Contraindicated**	**Contraindicated**	**Contraindicated**	Use if indicated	Use if indicated	Use if indicated	Use if indicated
Hepatitis A	Use if indicated	Use if indicated	Use if indicated	Use if indicated	Use if indicated	Use if indicated	Recommended[2]
Hepatitis B	Recommended	Recommended	Recommended	Recommended	Recommended	Recommended	Recommended
Influenza	Recommended[3]	Recommended	Recommended	Recommended	Recommended	Recommended	Recommended
Measles, mumps, rubella	**Contraindicated**	Recommended[4]	**Contraindicated**	Recommended	Recommended	Recommended	Recommended
Meningo-coccus	Use if indicated	Use if indicated	Use if indicated	Recommended[2]	Use if indicated	Use if indicated	Use if indicated
Poliovirus vaccine, IPV[5]	Use if indicated	Use if indicated	Use if indicated	Use if indicated	Use if indicated	Use if indicated	Use if indicated
Poliovirus vaccine, OPV[5]	Use if indicated	**Contraindicated**	**Contraindicated**	Use if indicated	Use if indicated	Use if indicated	Use if indicated
Pneumo-coccus[2]	Use if indicated	Recommended	Recommended	Recommended	Recommended	Recommended	Recommended
Rabies	Use if indicated	Use if indicated	Use if indicated	Use if indicated	Use if indicated	Use if indicated	Use if indicated

Tetanus/ diphtheria[2]	Recommended	Recommended	Recommended	Recommended	Recommended	Recommended	Recommended
Typhoid, inactivated and Vi[6]	Use if indicated	Use if indicated	Use if indicated	Use if indicated	Use if indicated	Use if indicated	Use if indicated
Typhoid, Ty21a	Use if indicated	**Contraindicated**	**Contraindicated**	Use if indicated	Use if indicated	Use if indicated	Use if indicated
Varicella	**Contraindicated**	**Contraindicated**	**Contraindicated**	Recommended	Recommended	Recommended	Recommended
Vaccinia	**Contraindicated**	**Contraindicated**	**Contraindicated**	Use if indicated	Use if indicated	Use if indicated	Use if indicated

Adapted from Centers for Disease Control and Prevention. Immunization of health-care workers. Recommendations of the Advisory Committee on Immunization Practices (ACIP) and the Hospital Infection Control Practices Advisory Committee (HICPAC). *MMWR Morb Mortal Wkly Rep* 1997;46 (RR-18):30.

[1]Severe immunosuppression can be caused by congenital immunodeficiency, leukemia, lymphoma, generalized malignancy, or therapy with alkylating agents, antimetabolites, ionizing radiation, or large amounts of corticosteroids.

[2]Recommendation is based on the person's underlying condition rather than occupation.

[3]Women who will be in the second or third trimester of pregnancy (≥14 weeks' gestation) during the influenza season.

[4]Contraindicated in HIV-infected persons who have evidence of severe immunosuppression.

[5]Vaccination is recommended for unvaccinated health-care workers who have close contact with patients who may be excreting wild polioviruses. Primary vaccination with IPV is recommended because the risk for vaccine-associated paralysis after administration of OPV is higher among adults than among children. Health-care workers who have had a primary series of OPV or IPV and who are directly involved with the provision of care to patients who may be excreting poliovirus may receive another dose of either IPV or OPV. Any suspected case of poliomyelitis should be investigated immediately. If evidence suggests transmission of wild poliovirus, control measures to contain further transmission should be instituted immediately, including an OPV vaccination campaign.

[6]Capsular polysaccharide parenteral vaccine.

Work Restrictions for Infected Health-Care Workers (HCWs) Exposed to Certain Vaccine-Preventable Diseases

Disease	Work Restriction	Duration
Diphtheria		
Active	Exclude from duty	Until antimicrobial therapy is completed and 2 nasopharyngeal cultures obtained ≥24 hours apart are negative
Postexposure (susceptible HCWs; previously vaccinated HCWs who have not had a Td booster dose within the previous 5 years)	Exclude from duty	Same as active diphtheria
Asymptomatic carriers	Exclude from duty	Same as active diphtheria
Hepatitis A	Relieve from patient contact and food handling	7 days after onset of jaundice
Hepatitis B		
HCWs who do not perform exposure-prone invasive procedures	Standard precautions should always be observed; no restriction unless epidemiologically linked to transmission of infection	Standard precautions should always be observed
HCWs who perform exposure-prone invasive procedures	These HCWs should not perform exposure-prone invasive procedures until they have sought counsel from an expert review panel, which should review and recommend the procedures the worker can perform, taking into account the specific procedure as well as the skill and technique of the worker	Until HBeAg negative

Upper Respiratory Tract Infections	During particular seasons (e.g., during winter when influenza and RSV are prevalent), consider excluding personnel with acute febrile upper respiratory tract infections (including influenza) from care of high-risk patients	Until acute symptoms resolve
Measles		
Active	Exclude from duty	7 days after rash appears
Postexposure (susceptible personnel)	Exclude from duty	5th day after first exposure through 21st day after last exposure and/or 7 days after the rash appears
Mumps		
Active	Exclude from duty	9 days after onset of parotitis
Postexposure (susceptible personnel)	Exclude from duty	12th day after first exposure through 26th day after last exposure or 9 days after onset of parotitis
Pertussis		
Active	Exclude from duty	Beginning of catarrhal stage through third week after onset of paroxysms or until 5 days after start of effective antimicrobial therapy (page 181)

Table continued on following page

Disease	Work Restriction	Duration
Postexposure		
Symptomatic personnel	Exclude from duty	5 days after start of effective antimicrobial therapy (page 181)
Asymptomatic personnel	No restriction if HCW taking antimicrobial prophylactic therapy	
Rubella		
Active	Exclude from duty	5 days after the rash appears
Postexposure (susceptible personnel)	Exclude from duty	7th day after first exposure through 21st day after last exposure and/or 5 days after rash appears
Varicella		
Active	Exclude from duty	Until all lesions dry and crust
Postexposure (susceptible personnel)	Exclude from duty	8th day (AAP) or 10th day (ACIP) after first exposure through 21st day (28th day if VZIG administered) after the last exposure; if varicella occurs, until all lesions dry and crust

Zoster		
Localized (immunocompetent host)	Cover lesions; restrict from care of patients susceptible to varicella and at increased risk for complications of varicella (e.g., neonates and immunocompromised persons of any age)	Same as varicella
Postexposure (susceptible personnel)	Restrict from patient contact	Same as varicella

Adapted from Centers for Disease Control and Prevention. Immunization of health-care workers. Recommendations of the Advisory Committee on Immunization Practices (ACIP) and the Hospital Infection Control Practices Advisory Committee (HICPAC). *MMWR Morb Mortal Wkly Rep* 1997;46 (RR-18):33–34; Centers for Disease Control and Prevention. Recommendations for preventing transmission of human immunodeficiency virus and hepatitis B virus to patients during exposure-prone invasive procedures. *MMWR Morb Mortal Wkly Rep* 1991;40 (RR-8):1–8; Centers for Disease Control and Prevention. Guidelines for isolation precautions in hospitals. Recommendations of the Hospital Infection Control Practices Advisory Committee (HICPAC) and the National Center for Infectious Diseases. *Infect Control Hosp Epidemiol* 1996;17:53–80; Williams WW: CDC guideline for infection control in hospital personnel. *Infect Control* 1983;4(suppl):326–349.

Immunization of Patients with Altered Immunity

Immunization of Immunocompromised Infants and Children

Vaccine	Routine (Not Immuno-compromised)	HIV Infection/ AIDS	Severely Immuno-compromised[1] (Non–HIV Related)	Asplenia	Renal Failure	Diabetes
Routine Childhood Immunizations						
DTP (DTaP/DT/T/Td)	Recommended	Recommended	Recommended	Recommended	Recommended	Recommended
Haemophilus influenzae type b	Recommended	Recommended	Recommended	Recommended	Recommended	Recommended
Hepatitis B	Recommended	Recommended	Recommended	Recommended	Recommended	Recommended
MMR (MR/M/R)	Recommended	Recommended/ considered[2]	**Contraindicated**	Recommended	Recommended	Recommended
Polio						
OPV	Recommended	**Contraindicated**	**Contraindicated**	Recommended	Recommended	Recommended
IPV	Recommended	Recommended	Recommended	Use if indicated	Use if indicated	Use if indicated
Varicella	Recommended	**Contraindicated**	**Contraindicated**	**Contraindicated**	Use if indicated	Recommended
Other Childhood Immunizations						
Influenza[3]	Use if indicated	Recommended	Recommended	Recommended	Recommended	Recommended
Pneumococcus[4]	Use if indicated	Recommended	Recommended	Recommended	Recommended	Recommended

Adapted from Centers for Disease Control and Prevention. Recommendations of the Advisory Committee on Immunization Practices (ACIP): use of vaccines and immune globulins in persons with altered immunocompetence. *MMWR Morb Mortal Wkly Rep* 1993;42 (RR-4):15.

[1]Severe immunosuppression can be the result of congenital immunodeficiency, HIV infection, leukemia, lymphoma, aplastic anemia, generalized malignancy, or therapy with alkylating agents, antimetabolites, radiation, or large amounts of corticosteroids. See discussion of MMR.

[2]Measles vaccination is recommended for HIV-infected persons without evidence of measles immunity who are not severely immunocompromised (CD4+ >200/μL for persons ≥6 years of age, >500/μL for children 1–5 years of age, or >750/μL for children <12 months of age). Severely immunocompromised HIV-infected persons (CD4+ <200/μL for persons ≥6 years of age, <500/μL for children 1–5 years of age, or <750/μL for children <12 months of age) who are exposed to measles should receive immune globulin, regardless of prior vaccination status.

[3]Not recommended for infants <6 months of age.

[4]Recommended for persons ≥2 years of age.

IMMUNIZATION SCHEDULE FOR HIV-EXPOSED OR HIV-INFECTED CHILDREN[1]

Age ▶ Vaccine[1] ▼	Birth	1 mo	2 mo	4 mo	6 mo	12 mo	15 mo	18 mo	24 mo	4–6 yr	11–12 yr	14–16 yr
⬇ Recommendations for these vaccines are the same as those for immunocompetent children ⬇												
Hepatitis B[2,3]	Hep B-1											
		Hep B-2			Hep B-3						Hep B	
Diphtheria, tetanus, pertussis[4]			DTaP or DTP	DTaP or DTP	DTaP or DTP		DTaP or DTP			DTaP or DTP	Td	
Haemophilus influenzae type b[5]			Hib	Hib	Hib	Hib						
⬇ Recommendations for these vaccines differ from those for immunocompetent children ⬇												
Polio[6]			IPV	IPV		IPV				IPV		
Measles, mumps, rubella[7]						MMR	MMR					
Influenza[8]					Influenza (a dose is required every year)							
Streptococcus pneumoniae[9]									Pneumococcal			
Varicella						**CONTRAINDICATED in *all* HIV-infected persons**						

Adapted from Centers for Disease Control and Prevention. 1997 USPHS/IDSA guidelines for the prevention of opportunistic infections in persons infected with human immunodeficiency virus. *MMWR Morb Mortal Wkly Rep* 1997:46 (RR-12):34–35.

[1]Modified from the immunization schedule for immunocompetent children (page 2). This schedule also applies to children born to HIV-infected mothers whose HIV infection status has not been determined. Once a child is known not to be HIV infected, the schedule for immunocompetent children applies. This schedule indicates the recommended age for routine administration of currently licensed childhood vaccines; vaccines are listed under the ages for which they are routinely recommended. Bars indicate the range of acceptable ages for vaccination. Catch-up immunization should be done during any visit when feasible. Shaded oval indicates catch-up vaccination; at 11–12 years of age, hepatitis B vaccine should be administered to children not previously vaccinated. Combination vaccines (page 74) may be used whenever any components of the combination are indicated and its other components are not contraindicated. Providers should consult the manufacturers' package inserts for detailed recommendations.

[2]***Infants born to HBsAg-negative mothers*** should receive 2.5 μg of Merck vaccine (Recombivax HB) or 10 μg of SmithKline Beecham vaccine (Engerix-B). The second dose should be administered at least 1 month after the first dose. The third dose should be given at least 2 months after the second dose, but not before 6 months of age.

Infants born to HBsAg-positive mothers should receive 0.5 mL hepatitis B immune globulin (HBIG) within 12 hours of birth and either 5 μg of Merck vaccine (Recombivax HB) or 10 μg of SmithKline Beecham vaccine (Engerix-B) at a separate site. The second dose is recommended at 1–2 months of age and the third dose at 6 months of age (page 205).

Infants born to mothers whose HBsAg status is unknown should receive either 5 μg of Merck vaccine (Recombivax HB) or 10 μg of SmithKline Beecham vaccine (Engerix-B) within 12 hours of birth. The second dose of vaccine is recommended at 1–2 months of age and the third dose at 6 months of age. Blood should be drawn at the time of delivery to determine the mother's HBsAg status; if it is positive, the infant should receive HBIG as soon as possible (not later than 1 week of age). The dosage and timing of subsequent vaccine doses should be based on the mother's HBsAg status (page 59).

Legend continued on following page

[3]Children and adolescents who have not been vaccinated against hepatitis B in infancy may begin the series during any visit. Those who have not previously received 3 doses of hepatitis B vaccine should initiate or complete the series during the routine visit to a health-care provider at 11–12 years of age, and unvaccinated older adolescents should be vaccinated whenever possible. The second dose should be administered at least 1 month after the first dose, and the third dose should be administered at least 4 months after the first dose and at least 2 months after the second dose.

[4]DTaP (diphtheria and tetanus toxoids and acellular pertussis vaccine) is the preferred vaccine for all doses in the vaccination series, including completion of the series in children who have received 1 or more doses of DTP (diphtheria and tetanus toxoids and whole-cell pertussis vaccine). Whole-cell DTP is an acceptable alternative to DTaP. The fourth dose (DTaP or DTP) may be administered as early as 12 months of age if 6 months have elapsed since the third dose and if the child is unlikely to return at 15–18 months of age. Td (tetanus and diphtheria toxoids, for adult use) is recommended at 11–12 years of age if at least 5 years have elapsed since the last dose of DTP, DTaP, or DT (tetanus and diphtheria toxoids, for pediatric use). Subsequent routine Td (tetanus and diphtheria toxoids, for adult use) boosters are recommended every 10 years.

[5]Three *H. influenzae* type b (Hib) conjugate vaccines are licensed for infant use. If PRP-OMP (PedvaxHIB [Merck]) is administered at 2 and 4 months of age, a dose at 6 months is not required. After completing the primary series, any Hib conjugate vaccine may be used as a booster.

[6]Inactivated poliovirus vaccine (IPV) is the only polio vaccine recommended for HIV-infected persons and their household contacts. Although the third dose of IPV is generally administered at 12–18 months of age, the third dose of IPV has been approved to be administered as early as 6 months of age. Oral poliovirus vaccine (OPV) should *not* be administered to HIV-infected persons or their household contacts.

[7]MMR should not be administered to severely immunocompromised children (see table below). Asymptomatic or symptomatic HIV-infected children without severe immunosuppression should routinely receive their first dose of MMR as soon as possible on reaching the first birthday. Consideration should be given to administering the second dose of MMR vaccine as soon as 1 month (i.e., a minimum of 28 days) after the first dose, rather than waiting until school entry.

Criteria for Severe Immunosuppression for HIV-infected Persons

	Age			
Cell Count	**<12 mo**	**1–5 yr**	**6–12 yr**	**≥13 yr**
Total CD4	<750/μL	<500/μL	<200/μL	<200/μL
or				
% CD4	<15%	<15%	<15%	<14%

[8]Influenza virus vaccine should be administered to all HIV-infected children >6 months of age each year. Children 6 months to 8 years of age who are receiving influenza vaccine for the first time should receive 2 doses of split-virus vaccine separated by at least 1 month. In subsequent years, a single dose of vaccine (split virus for persons ≤12 years of age, whole or split virus for persons >12 years of age) should be administered each year. The dose of vaccine for children 6–35 months of age is 0.25 mL; the dose for children ≥3 years of age is 0.5 mL (page 81).

[9]The 23-valent pneumococcal vaccine should be administered to HIV-infected children at 24 months of age. Revaccination should generally be offered to HIV-infected children vaccinated 3–5 years (children aged ≤10 years of age at revaccination) or >5 years (children aged >10 years of age at revaccination) earlier (page 85).

Immunization of Immunocompromised Adults

Vaccine	Routine (Not Immunocompromised)	HIV Infection/ AIDS	Severely Immunocompromised[1] (Non-HIV Related)	After Solid Organ Transplant or Long-term Immunosuppression Therapy
Routine Immunizations				
Td	Recommended	Recommended	Recommended	Recommended
Haemophilus influenzae type b	Not recommended	Considered	Recommended	Recommended
Hepatitis B	Use if indicated	Use if indicated	Use if indicated	Use if indicated
MMR (MR/M/R)	Use if indicated	Considered[2]	**Contraindicated**	**Contraindicated**
Polio				
OPV	Use if indicated	**Contraindicated**	**Contraindicated**	**Contraindicated**
IPV	Use if indicated	Use if indicated	Use if indicated	Use if indicated
Varicella	Not recommended	**Contraindicated**	**Contraindicated**	**Contraindicated**
Special-Use Immunizations				
Anthrax	Use if indicated	Use if indicated	Use if indicated	Use if indicated
BCG	Use if indicated	**Contraindicated**	**Contraindicated**	**Contraindicated**
Cholera	Use if indicated	Use if indicated	Use if indicated	Use if indicated
Hepatitis A	Use if indicated	Use if indicated	Use if indicated	Use if indicated
Influenza	Recommended if ≥65 years of age	Recommended	Recommended	Recommended

Meningococcus	Use if indicated	Use if indicated	Use if indicated	Use if indicated
Plague	Use if indicated	Use if indicated	Use if indicated	Use if indicated
Pneumococcus	Recommended if ≥65 years of age	Recommended	Recommended	Recommended
Rabies	Use if indicated	Use if indicated	Use if indicated	Use if indicated
Typhoid, Ty21a	Use if indicated	**Contraindicated**	**Contraindicated**	**Contraindicated**
Typhoid, inactivated and Vi	Use if indicated	Use if indicated	Use if indicated	Use if indicated
Yellow fever[3]	Use if indicated	**Contraindicated**	**Contraindicated**	**Contraindicated**

Vaccine	**Asplenia**	**Renal Failure**	**Diabetes**	**Alcoholism and Alcoholic Cirrhosis**
Routine Immunizations				
Td	Recommended	Recommended	Recommended	Recommended
Haemophilus influenzae type b	Recommended	Use if indicated	Use if indicated	Use if indicated
Hepatitis B	Use if indicated	Recommended[4]	Use if indicated	Use if indicated
MMR (MR/M/R)	Use if indicated	Use if indicated	Use if indicated	Use if indicated
Poliomyelitis				
OPV	Use if indicated	Use if indicated	Use if indicated	Use if indicated
IPV	Use if indicated	Use if indicated	Use if indicated	Use if indicated
Varicella	**Contraindicated**	Use if indicated	Use if indicated	Use if indicated
Special-Use Immunizations				
Anthrax	Use if indicated	Use if indicated	Use if indicated	Use if indicated
BCG	Use if indicated	Use if indicated	Use if indicated	Use if indicated
Cholera	Use if indicated	Use if indicated	Use if indicated	Use if indicated

Table continued on following page

Vaccine	Asplenia	Renal Failure	Diabetes	Alcoholism and Alcoholic Cirrhosis
Hepatitis A	Use if indicated	Use if indicated	Use if indicated	Recommended
Influenza	Recommended	Recommended	Recommended	Recommended
Meningococcus	Recommended	Use if indicated	Use if indicated	Use if indicated
Plague	Use if indicated	Use if indicated	Use if indicated	Use if indicated
Pneumococcus	Recommended	Recommended	Recommended	Recommended
Rabies	Use if indicated	Use if indicated	Use if indicated	Use if indicated
Typhoid, Ty21a	Use if indicated	Use if indicated	Use if indicated	Use if indicated
Typhoid, inactivated and Vi	Use if indicated	Use if indicated	Use if indicated	Use if indicated
Yellow fever[3]	Use if indicated	Use if indicated	Use if indicated	Use if indicated

Adapted from Centers for Disease Control and Prevention. Recommendations of the Advisory Committee on Immunization Practices (ACIP): use of vaccines and immune globulins in persons with altered immunocompetence. *MMWR Morb Mortal Wkly Rep* 1993;42 (RR-4):16–17.

[1]Severe immunosuppression can be the result of congenital immunodeficiency, HIV infection, leukemia, lymphoma, aplastic anemia, generalized malignancy, or therapy with alkylating agents, antimetabolites, radiation, or large amounts of corticosteroids.

[2]Measles vaccination is recommended for asymptomatic and symptomatic HIV-infected persons without evidence of measles immunity who are not severely immunocompromised (for persons ≥13 years of age, CD4 cell count ≥200/μL and ≥14% of total lymphocytes). Severely immunocompromised HIV-infected persons (for persons ≥13 years of age, CD4 cell count <200/μL or <14% of total lymphocytes) who are exposed to measles should receive immune globulin, regardless of prior vaccination status.

[3]Yellow fever vaccine should be considered for patients when exposure to yellow fever cannot be avoided.

[4]Patients with renal failure on dialysis should have their anti-HBs response tested after vaccination, and those found not to respond should be revaccinated.

Vaccine Summaries

ROUTINE IMMUNIZATIONS FOR CHILDREN

DTaP/DTP[1–3] Vaccines

Routine Indications

Routine use[1–3]

- *Children <7 years of age:* universal immunization of infants and children beginning at 6–8 weeks of age[2]
  - Immunization beginning as early as 4 weeks of age in areas with high endemicity and during outbreaks
- Postexposure prophylaxis for tetanus for certain wounds in children who have not completed the primary DTaP/DTP schedule (page 186)
- *Adolescents and adults*: DTaP and DTP are not used in adolescents and adults

International travel

- All travelers should be vaccinated with DTaP/DTP/DT/Td appropriate for age

Contraindications

- An immediate anaphylactic reaction to a previous dose of DTP/DTaP/DT/Td

---

[1]DTP is also known as DTwP (whole-cell pertussis). DTaP (diphtheria and tetanus toxoids and acellular pertussis vaccine) is the preferred vaccine for all doses in the vaccination series, including completion of the series in children who have received 1 or more doses of whole-cell DTP vaccine.

[2]In the United States, DTaP is the preferred vaccine for all doses in the vaccination schedule, including completion of the series in children who have received 1 or more doses of whole-cell DTP vaccine, and for the fourth and fifth booster doses in children who received 3 doses of whole-cell DTP vaccine. Whole-cell DTP is an acceptable alternative to DTaP. The fourth dose (DTaP or DTP) may be administered as early as 12 months of age if 6 months have elapsed since the third dose and if the child is unlikely to return at 15–18 months of age.

[3]Combination vaccines (page 74) of DTaP/DTP and Hib include Tetramune (DTP/HbOC), which is approved for all DTP doses, and TriHIBit, which is PRP-T (ActHIB) reconstituted with DTaP produced by Pasteur Mérieux Connaught (Tripedia) for the booster (fourth dose) of DTP in children ≥15 months of age.

- Allergy to a vaccine component
- Moderate or severe illnesses with or without a fever
- History of culture-confirmed pertussis (use DT)
- Encephalopathy[4] not from another identifiable cause occurring within 7 days of administration of DTaP or DTP
- *For DTP only:*
  - Age ≥7 years of age (use DT or Td; DTaP is not contraindicated, but there are no current recommendations for immunization of adolescents or adults with any pertussis vaccine)

Precautions[5]

- Fever of ≥40.5°C (≥105°F) that is not attributed to another identifiable cause occurring within 48 hours after administration of a previous dose of DTP
- Collapse or shocklike state (i.e., a hypotonic-hyporesponsive episode) occurring within 48 hours after administration of a previous dose of DTP
- Convulsions with or without fever occurring within 3 days after administration of a previous dose of DTP
- Persistent, inconsolable crying lasting ≥3 hours and occurring within 48 hours after administration of a previous dose of DTP

Not Contraindications

- Soreness, redness, or swelling at the site of a previous DTP vaccination
- Temperature <40.5°C (<105°F) occurring within 48 hours after administration of a previous dose of DTP

---

[4]Whether and when to administer DTP to children with proven or suspected underlying neurological disorders should be decided on an individual basis. Encephalopathies include major alterations in consciousness; unresponsiveness; generalized or focal seizures that persist more than a few hours with failure to recover within 24 hours; or other generalized or focal neurological signs.

[5]These events, which are not associated with permanent sequelae, were once considered absolute contraindications but there may be circumstances, such as with a high incidence of pertussis, that the potential benefits outweigh possible risks.

- Mild, acute illness with low-grade fever or mild diarrheal illness affecting an otherwise healthy child
- Current antimicrobial therapy or the convalescent phase of an acute illness
- Recent exposure to an infectious disease
- Prematurity (The usual chronological age from birth should be used to initiate vaccination of premature infants. The full dosage of vaccine should be used.)
- History of allergies or relatives with allergies
- Family history of convulsions[6]
- Family history of sudden infant death syndrome (SIDS)
- Family history of an adverse event following DTP administration

Administration

- 0.5 mL intramuscularly in the anterolateral aspect of the mid-thigh for children <24 months of age or the deltoid muscle for older children (Do not administer into the gluteal region.)

---

[6]Acetaminophen (every 4 hours) or ibuprofen (every 6–8 hours) given before administering DTP and thereafter for 24 hours should be considered for children with a personal or family history of convulsions in siblings or parents.

Adverse Events Associated with Diphtheria and Tetanus Toxoids and Pertussis Vaccines[1]

		DTaP Vaccines		
Reaction	**DTP**	**Acel-Imune**	**Infanrix**	**Tripedia**
Local Reactions				
Pain	40%	4%	11%	10%
Swelling	61%	16%	30%	20%
Erythema	73%	26%	39%	33%
Systemic Reactions				
Fever >101°F (>38.3°C)	16%	3%	3%	5%
Fussiness	42%	14%	15%	19%
Drowsiness	62%	41%	47%	42%
Anorexia	35%	25%	19%	22%
Vomiting	14%	13%	13%	7%
Persistent, inconsolable crying (≥3 hours)	1%			
Fever ≥105°F (≥40.5°C)	1 per 330 doses			
Collapse (hypotonic-hyporesponsive episode)	1 per 1750 doses			
Convulsions (with or without fever)	1 per 1750 doses			

Adapted from Centers for Disease Control and Prevention. Pertussis vaccination: use of acellular pertussis vaccines among infants and young children. Recommendations of the Advisory Committee on Immunization Practices (ACIP). *MMWR Morb Mortal Wkly Rep* 1997;46(RR-7):42.

[1]Percentage of infants with the indicated reaction by the third evening after any dose of pertussis vaccine administered at ages 2, 4, and 6 months.

Licensed Uses of DTaP and DTP Vaccines

Trade Name	Manufacturer	Date Approved	Licensed Uses
DTaP Vaccines			
Acel-Imune	Wyeth-Lederle	December 1996	All 5 doses (2, 4, 6, 15–18 months, and 4–6 years)
Certiva	North American Vaccine/Ross	July 1998	First 4 doses (2, 4, 6, and 15–18 months) May be used for the fifth dose in children who have received ≥1 dose of whole-cell DTP
Infanrix	SmithKline Beecham	January 1997	First 4 doses (2, 4, 6, and 15–18 months)[1]
Tripedia	Connaught	July 1996	First 4 doses (2, 4, 6, and 15–18 months)[1]
TriHIBit (ActHIB[2] [PRP-T] reconstituted with Tripedia [DTaP])	Connaught	September 1996	Fourth dose only (15–18 months)[3]
DTP Vaccines			
Tetramune (HibTITER [HbOC]) and Tri-Immunol (DTwP)	Lederle	March 1993	All 5 doses (2, 4, 6, 15–18 months, and 4–6 years)

[1]A fifth dose will be required; FDA approval for use for the fifth dose is pending as of September 1, 1998.

[2]ActHIB is identical to OmniHIB.

[3]FDA approval for use for the first 3 doses is pending as of September 1, 1998.

DT/Td Vaccines

Routine Indications

Routine use

DT (tetanus and diphtheria toxoids, absorbed, for pediatric use)

- *Children <7 years of age*:
  - Primary diphtheria and pertussis vaccination of individuals for whom pertussis vaccination is contraindicated (e.g., children ≥7 years of age and adults, especially pregnant women)
  - Postexposure prophylaxis for tetanus for certain wounds in children ≥7 years of age (page 186)

Td (tetanus and diphtheria toxoids, absorbed, for adult use)

- *Adolescents*: at 11–12 years of age if not vaccinated within the previous 5 years
- *Adults* (including *health-care workers*): booster doses every 10 years throughout life (especially for pregnant women)
- Postexposure prophylaxis for tetanus for certain wounds in children >7 years of age, adolescents, and adults (page 186)

International travel

- All travelers should be vaccinated with DTaP/DTP/DT/Td appropriate for age

Contraindications

- Encephalopathy[1] not from another identifiable cause occurring within 7 days of administration of DTaP/DTP/DT/Td
- An immediate anaphylactic reaction to a previous dose of DTaP/DTP/DT/Td
- Allergy to a vaccine component
- Moderate or severe illnesses with or without a fever

[1]Whether and when to administer DTP to children with proven or suspected underlying neurological disorders should be decided on an individual basis. Encephalopathies include major alterations in consciousness; unresponsiveness; generalized or focal seizures that persist more than a few hours with failure to recover within 24 hours; or other generalized or focal neurological signs.

Not Contraindications

- Soreness, redness, or swelling at the site of DTP vaccination
- Temperature <40.5°C (<105°F) occurring within 48 hours after administration of a previous dose of DTP
- Mild, acute illness with low-grade fever or mild diarrheal illness affecting an otherwise healthy child
- Current antimicrobial therapy or the convalescent phase of an acute illness
- Recent exposure to an infectious disease
- History of allergies or relatives with allergies
- Family history of convulsions[2]
- Family history of sudden infant death syndrome (SIDS)
- Family history of an adverse event following DTP administration
- Pregnancy or breast-feeding

Administration

- 0.5 mL intramuscularly in the anterolateral aspect of the mid-thigh for children <24 months of age or the deltoid muscle for older children (DT for children <7 years of age, dT for children ≥7 years of age), adolescents (dT), and adults (dT) (Do not administer into the gluteal region.)

---

[2]Acetaminophen (every 4 hours) or ibuprofen (every 6–8 hours) given before administering DTP and thereafter for 24 hours should be considered for children with a personal or family history of convulsions in siblings or parents.

Constituents of DTaP/DTP/DT/Td Vaccines (per 0.5 mL dose)

Vaccine	Diphtheria Toxoid	Tetanus Toxoid	Pertussis Component
DTaP Vaccines			
Pasteur Mérieux Connaught (Tripedia)	6.7 Lf	5 Lf	Pertussis toxin (PT), inactivated 23.4 μg Filamentous hemagglutinin (FHA) 23.4 μg
SmithKline Beecham (Infanrix)	17 Lf	10 Lf	Pertussis toxin (PT), inactivated 25 μg Filamentous hemagglutinin (FHA) 25 μg
Wyeth-Lederle (Acel-Imune)	7.5 Lf	5 Lf	300 HA units (40-60 μg of protein) Filamentous hemagglutinin (FHA) 86% Pertussis toxin (PT), inactivated 8% Pertactin 8% Fimbria type 2
Chiron-Biocine[1]	25 Lf	10 Lf	Pertussis toxin (PT), inactivated 5 μg Filamentous hemagglutinin (FHA) 2.5 μg Pertactin 2.5 μg
North American Vaccine/Ross (Certiva)	25 Lf	7 Lf	Pertussis toxin (PT), inactivated 40 μg
DTP Vaccines			
Connaught	6.5 Lf	5 Lf	4 units (whole cell)
Wyeth-Lederle (Tri-Immunol)	12.5 Lf	5 Lf	4 units (whole cell)
Massachusetts PHBL	10 Lf	5.5 Lf	4 units (whole cell)
Michigan BPI	10 Lf	5.5 Lf	4 units (whole cell)

DT Vaccines			
Connaught	6.6 Lf	5 Lf	None
Lederle	5 Lf	12.5 Lf	
Massachusetts PHBL	7.5 Lf	7.5 Lf	
Michigan BPI	Not provided	Not provided	
Sclavo	15 Lf	10 Lf	
Wyeth-Ayerst	10 Lf	5 Lf	
Td Vaccines			
Connaught	5 Lf	2 Lf	None
Lederle	5 Lf	2 Lf	
Massachusetts PHBL	2 Lf	2 Lf	
Sclavo	10 Lf	2 Lf	
Wyeth-Ayerst	5 Lf	2 Lf	

[1]FDA approval for licensure is pending as of September 1, 1998.

Haemophilus influenzae type b (Hib) Vaccines

Routine Indications

Routine use

- *Children*: universal immunization of infants and children beginning at 6–8 weeks of age
  - Unimmunized children <24 months of age with invasive *H. influenzae* disease[1] (initiate revaccination 1 month after onset of disease)
- *Adolescents* and *adults* (including *health-care workers*): routine Hib vaccination not recommended

High-risk groups

- Unimmunized children ≥5 years of age and adults with:
  - Functional or anatomical asplenia
  - Hematological neoplasms (administered 10–14 days before initiation of chemotherapy *or* 3 months after cessation of chemotherapy)
- Persons with HIV infection

International travel

- All travelers should be vaccinated with Hib appropriate for age

Contraindications

- An immediate anaphylactic reaction to a previous dose of any Hib vaccine
- Allergy to a vaccine component
- Moderate or severe illnesses with or without a fever

Not Contraindications

- History of invasive *H. influenzae* disease[1]

---

[1]Children who experience invasive Hib disease after receiving a dose of conjugate vaccine at ≥15 months of age or who completed a recommended Hib immunization before 15 months of age (i.e., a final dose at 12–14 months of age) have an increased incidence of IgG_2 deficiency and should be considered for immunological evaluation. The necessity for immunological evaluation of children who experience invasive Hib disease after receiving a dose of conjugate vaccine administered earlier than 12 months of age is uncertain.

  - Individuals <24 months of age with invasive *H. influenzae* disease have a poor antibody response and remain at risk and should be immunized
  - Individuals ≥24 months of age with invasive *H. influenzae* disease usually develop a protective immune response but may be immunized
- Pregnancy or breast-feeding

Administration

- 0.5 mL intramuscularly in the anterolateral aspect of the mid-thigh for children <24 months of age or the deltoid muscle for older children (Do not administer into the gluteal region.)
- In patients with coagulation disorders, PRP-T, 0.5 mL, may be given subcutaneously in the anterolateral aspect of the mid-thigh
- The three conjugate vaccines are considered interchangeable for primary as well as booster vaccination (If PRP-OMP is administered in a series with one of the other two Hib vaccines, the third dose of any of the three Hib vaccines is necessary at 6 months of age to complete the primary series.)

Schedule for Routine Administration

Vaccine[1]	2 Mo	4 Mo	6 Mo	12–15 Mo
PRP-OMP (PedvaxHIB [Merck])	Dose 1	Dose 2	*(not required)*	Booster
HbOC (HibTITER, Tetramune [DTP and Hib][1] [Lederle])	Dose 1	Dose 2	Dose 3	Booster
PRP-T[1] (ActHIB [Pasteur Mérieux Connaught]; OmniHIB [SmithKline Beecham])	Dose 1	Dose 2	Dose 3	Booster
PRP-D (ProHIBit [Pasteur Mérieux Connaught])	Not approved for children <15 mo of age; dose 1 at 15 mo			

[1]Combination vaccines (page 74) of DTaP/DTP and Hib include DTP/HbOC (Tetramune), which is approved for all DTP doses, and TriHIBit, which is PRP-T (ActHIB) reconstituted with DTaP produced by Pasteur Mérieux Connaught (Tripedia) for the booster (fourth dose) of DTP in children ≥15 months of age.

Schedule for Children with a Lapse in Hib Vaccination

Age at Presentation	Prior Vaccination History	Recommended Regimen
7–11 months	1 dose of OMP *or* 2 doses of HbOC or PRP-T	One dose of Hib at 7–11 months, with a booster dose at least 2 months later, at 12–15 months[1]
12–14 months	2 doses before 12 months	A single dose of any conjugate vaccine[2]
	1 dose before 12 months	Two additional doses of any licensed conjugate, separated by 2 months[2]
15–59 months	Any incomplete schedule	A single dose of any conjugate vaccine[2]

[1]If feasible, use the same vaccine for the dose at 7–11 months of age that was used for the dose given at 2–6 months of age. For the dose at 12–15 months of age, any conjugate vaccine can be used.

[2]The safety and efficacy of all licensed Hib conjugate vaccines are considered equivalent for children ≥12 months of age.

Constituents of Haemophilus influenzae *type b Conjugate Vaccines*[1]

Vaccine	Trade Name	Manufacturer	Protein Carrier	Polysaccharide Size and Amount	Linkage
PRP-OMP	PedvaxHIB	Merck	OMP (an outer membrane protein complex of group B *Neisseria meningitidis*)[1]	Medium; 15 μg/0.5 mL	Complex
HbOC	HibTITER	Lederle	Cross-reacting material (CRM_{197}; a nontoxic naturally occurring mutant of diphtheria toxin)[1]	Small; 10 μg/0.5 mL	Direct
	Tetramune (Hib and DTP)[2]	Lederle			
PRP-T	ActHIB[2]	Pasteur Mérieux Connaught	Tetanus toxoid[1]	Large; 10 μg/0.5 mL	6-carbon spacer
	OmniHIB[2]	SmithKline Beecham			
PRP-D	ProHIBit	Pasteur Mérieux Connaught	Diphtheria toxoid[1]	Medium; 25 μg/0.5 mL	6-carbon spacer

[1]Immunization with Hib vaccines using *N. meningitidis* (PRP-OMP), tetanus (PRP-T), or diphtheria (PRP-D) protein carriers is not immunogenic for the carrier proteins and is not a substitute for these vaccines.

[2]Combination vaccines (page 74) of DTaP/DTP and Hib include DTP/HbOC (Tetramune), which is approved for all DTP doses, and TriHIBit, which is PRP-T (ActHIB) reconstituted with DTaP produced by Pasteur Mérieux Connaught (Tripedia) for the booster (fourth dose) of DTP in children ≥15 months of age.

Hepatitis B Vaccines[1]

Routine Indications

Routine use

- *Children*: universal immunization of infants beginning at birth–2 months of age
  - Universal immunization of preterm infants of <35 weeks' gestation and <2 kg birth weight beginning at 2 months of age (begin vaccine series at birth if the mother is HbsAg positive [page 205]; begin vaccine series at 2 months of age if the mother is HbsAg negative)
- *Adolescents*: adolescents 11–12 years of age who have not been vaccinated previously and unvaccinated adolescents >12 years of age at increased risk of hepatitis B infection
- *Adults*: adults in high-risk groups who are at increased risk of hepatitis B infection or its complications

High-risk groups[2]

- Health-care workers (page 24)
  - Health-care workers and others with direct patient contact or exposure to blood or body fluids[2]
  - Staff (and residents) of institutions for developmentally disabled persons
  - Staff of nonresidential day care and school programs for developmentally disabled persons if attended by a known HBsAg-positive carrier
- Household contacts and sex partners of persons with acute hepatitis B or who have chronic HBV infection

---

[1]Prevaccination screening may be recommended for hepatitis B depending on the specific level of risk and/or likelihood of previous exposure to HBV.

[2]Health-care workers who have direct patient contact or exposure to blood or body fluids should be tested 1–2 months after completing vaccination to determine serological response. Persons with inadequate (<10 mIU/ml) or no anti-HBs are at risk for HBV infection and should be vaccinated with a second hepatitis B vaccination series. If the HCW has inadequate or no anti-HBs after a second vaccine series, the HCW is considered a nonresponder to hepatitis B vaccination. The HCW should be counseled that nonresponse most likely means that he or she is susceptible to hepatitis B infection. It is possible, however, that the HCW is chronically infected with HBV, and HBsAg testing is recommended.

- Immigrants/refugees/adopted children from areas of high hepatitis B endemicity (Asia, Pacific Islands, Sub-Saharan Africa, Amazon Basin, Eastern Europe, Middle East)
- Children born in the United States to, or who reside in households of, first-generation immigrants from countries where HBV is of high endemicity
  - Hemodialysis patients[3]
  - Hemophiliac patients and other recipients of certain blood products (clotting-factor concentrates)
- Residents (and staff) of institutions for developmentally disabled persons
- Persons who attend nonresidential day care and school programs for developmentally disabled persons if attended by a known HBsAg-positive carrier who behaves aggressively
- Persons at increased risk because of sexual or social habits
  - Sexually active heterosexual men and women who are diagnosed with a sexually transmitted disease, are prostitutes, or have a history of sexual activity with more than one sex partner in the previous 6 months
  - Men who have sex with men
  - Users of illicit injectable drugs
  - Inmates of long-term correctional institutions

International travel

- All children and adolescents ≤18 years of age should be immunized routinely

---

[3]Hemodialysis patients and immunocompromised patients (e.g., HIV-infected persons) should be tested 1–2 months after completing vaccination to determine serologic response. For patients who have responded to hepatitis B vaccination (≥10 mIU/mL), no HBsAg testing is needed, and anti-HBs should be performed annually with booster doses of hepatitis B vaccine to maintain anti-HBs concentrations of at least 10 mIU/mL. Patients with inadequate (<10 mIU/mL) or no anti-HBs are at risk for HBV infection and should be revaccinated with 1 or more additional doses of hepatitis B vaccine. Postvaccination anti-HBs testing should follow 1–2 months later. Until the patient is documented to have an adequate response, monthly HBsAg testing should be performed. If the patient continues with low or no anti-HBs and a total of 6 doses of Recombivax HB or 8 doses of Engerix-B vaccine have been given, the patient is considered a nonresponder to hepatitis B vaccination. Monthly HBsAg testing should be continued, and anti-HBs testing should be performed every 6 months.

- Adult international travelers who will live for more than 6 months in areas of high HBV endemicity (Southeast Asia, Africa, the Middle East, the islands of the South and Western Pacific, and the Amazon region of South America) and who will have close contact with the local population
- Adult travelers who are likely to have contact with blood from or sexual contact with residents of areas with high levels of endemic disease

Possible Indications

- Individuals who live or work in environments with a high likelihood of transmission of hepatitis B:
  - Teachers of young children
  - Day care workers
  - Residents and staff in institutional (e.g., nursing home) settings
- Individuals who live or work in environments in which hepatitis B transmission may occur
  - College students
  - Military personnel

Contraindications

- An immediate anaphylactic reaction to a previous dose of any hepatitis B vaccine
- Allergy to a vaccine component
  - History of anaphylactic reaction to common baker's yeast
- Moderate or severe illnesses with or without a fever

Not Contraindications

- Pregnancy or breast-feeding
- The vaccine produces neither therapeutic nor adverse effects in hepatitis B virus–infected persons

Administration

Doses and Schedules of Hepatitis B Vaccines

	Vaccine					
	Engerix-B[1]		Recombivax HB[1]		Comvax[2]	
	Dose		Dose		Dose	
Group	**μg**	**mL**	**μg**	**mL**	**μg**	**mL**
Infants of HBV-carrier mothers	10	0.5	5	0.5	Not approved	
Other infants and children <11 years of age	10	0.5	5	0.5	5	0.5
Children and adolescents 11–19 years of age	20	1	5	0.5	Not approved	
Adults >19 years of age	20	1	10	1	Not approved	
Dialysis and other immunocompromised persons	40	2[3]	40	1[4]	Not approved	

[1]Both vaccines are routinely administered intramuscularly in a 3-dose series at 0, 1, and 6 months. Engerix-B has also been licensed for a 4-dose series administered at 0, 1, 2, and 12 months.

[2]Comvax combines PedvaxHIB (*H. influenzae* type b conjugate [PRP-OMP], 7.5 μg) and Recombivax HB (hepatitis B, 5 μg) vaccines (page 74) for administration at 2 months, 4 months, and 12–15 months of age. Comvax should not be administered to infants <6 weeks of age. Comvax may be administered to infants given 1 dose of hepatitis B at or shortly after birth.

[3]Special formulation for dialysis patients.

[4]Two 1-mL doses administered at one site, in a 4-dose schedule at 0, 1, 2, and 6 months.

Measles, Mumps, and Rubella (MMR) Vaccines

Routine Indications

Routine use

- *Children*: universal immunization of infants and children[1] beginning at 12 months of age, with the second dose recommended at 4–6 years of age[2]
- *Adolescents*: immunization of adolescents not vaccinated previously with 2 doses of measles vaccine at ≥12 months of age[1,2]; those who have not previously received the second dose should complete the schedule no later than the 11- to 12-year visit
- *Adults*: adults born during or after 1957 without documentation of measles vaccine at ≥12 months of age

High-risk groups

- All *health-care workers*[3] (page 24)

International travel

- All international travelers (including travelers on cruise ships), particularly women of childbearing age
- Cruise ship crew members lacking documented immunity to rubella

Contraindications

- An immediate anaphylactic reaction to a previous dose of any measles, mumps, or rubella vaccine
- Allergy to a vaccine component

---

[1]Including HIV-infected persons (asymptomatic and symptomatic) who are not severely immunocompromised (page 39) if vaccination is otherwise indicated.

[2]The second measles dose is not a booster dose but is intended to overcome vaccine failure and to ensure that all children receive at least 1 dose of vaccine. The second dose of MMR is recommended routinely at 4–6 years of age but may be administered during any visit if at least 1 month has elapsed since receipt of the first dose and both doses are administered at or after 12 months of age.

[3]All HCWs (i.e., medical or nonmedical, paid or volunteer, full-time or part-time, student or nonstudent, with or without patient-care responsibilities) who work in facilities that provide health care to patients (i.e., inpatient or outpatient, public or private) should be immune to measles, rubella, and varicella. Facilities that provide care exclusively for elderly patients who are at minimal risk for measles and rubella and complications of these diseases are a possible exception.

  - History of anaphylactic reaction to neomycin or to gelatin or gelatin-containing products
- Moderate or severe acute illnesses with or without a fever
- Thrombocytopenia occurring within 6 weeks of a previous dose of vaccine
- Pregnancy; women should be counseled to avoid pregnancy for 3 months after administration of MMR or other rubella-containing vaccines or for 30 days after administration of monovalent measles or mumps vaccines
- Altered immunocompetence
  - Hematological and solid tumors
  - Primary immunodeficiency
  - Long-term immunosuppressive therapy, including high-dose corticosteroids (≥2 mg/kg/day *or* ≥20 mg/day daily or on alternate days for ≥14 days within the preceding month)
  - Severely immunocompromised HIV-infected persons (page 39)

Precautions[4]

- Persons with a history of thrombocytopenia or thrombocytopenic purpura
- Women should be counseled to avoid pregnancy for 3 months after administration of MMR or other rubella-containing vaccines or for 30 days after administration of monovalent measles or mumps vaccines
- Recent immune globulin administration[5,6] (page 112)

---

[4]No data exist to substantiate the theoretical risk of a suboptimal immune response from the administration of OPV and MMR within 30 days of each other.

[5]If an immune globulin is administered in the interval before vaccination is recommended (page 112), the recipient should be revaccinated at or after the appropriate interval unless serological testing indicates that measles-specific antibodies were induced.

[6]Postpartum administration of MMR or rubella vaccine to women who are susceptible to rubella should not be delayed because anti-Rh_o(D) immune globulin or any other blood product was administered during the last trimester of pregnancy or at delivery. Such rubella-susceptible women should be vaccinated immediately after delivery and tested at least 3 months later to ensure that they are immune to rubella and measles.

- Immune globulin products should not be administered for at least 2 weeks after vaccination[6]
- Persons with a history of anaphylactic reactions following egg ingestion should be vaccinated with caution (page 114)
- Measles vaccination may temporarily suppress tuberculin (TB) skin test reactivity[7]
- If varicella vaccine is not given at the same time, MMR and varicella vaccine should be administered at least 30 days apart

Not Contraindications[4]

- Mild acute illnesses with or without a fever
- Tuberculosis or positive TB skin test
- Simultaneous or recent TB skin test[6]
- Breast-feeding
- Pregnancy of the mother (or another household member) of the recipient
- Immunodeficient family member or household contact
- Short-term (<2 weeks) low- to moderate-dose systemic corticosteroid therapy, topical steroid therapy, long-term alternate-day therapy with low to moderate doses of short-acting corticosteroids, and intraarticular, bursal, or tendon injections of corticosteroids
- Patients with leukemia in remission who have not received chemotherapy for at least 3 months
- HIV-infected persons who are not severely immunocompromised (page 38)
- Nonanaphylactic reactions to eggs or neomycin
- Anaphylactic hypersensitivity to eggs or egg proteins
- Personal or family history of seizures

Administration

- 0.5 mL subcutaneously

---

[7]If tuberculin skin testing is indicated and cannot be done the day of MMR vaccination, the skin test should be postponed 4–6 weeks.

Poliovirus (IPV and OPV)

INACTIVATED POLIOVIRUS VACCINE (IPV or eIPV)

Routine Indications

Routine use

- *Children*:
  - Universal immunization of children beginning at 6–8 weeks of age, using either the sequential IPV/OPV schedule or the IPV-only schedule (page 67)
  - Infants of HIV-infected mothers (beginning at 2 months of age and continuing until the infant is known not to be HIV infected)
  - Symptomatic and asymptomatic HIV-exposed or HIV-infected children (until known not to be HIV infected)
  - Children with compromised immunity who are unimmunized or partially immunized
  - Children whose guardians refuse OPV
- *Adolescents and adults:* (Adults ≥18 years of age living in the United States who never received or completed a primary series of polio vaccine do not need to be vaccinated unless otherwise indicated.)
  - Unvaccinated adults in households (or other close contacts) of children who will be receiving oral poliovirus vaccine
  - Persons in communities or population groups experiencing polio disease
  - Laboratory workers who handle specimens that may contain polioviruses
- *Health-care workers* directly providing care to patients who may be excreting poliovirus

International travel

- Travelers to areas or countries where poliomyelitis is epidemic or endemic
- IPV, OPV, or sequential IPV/OPV for children
- IPV for unimmunized or partially immunized adults
- A once-per-lifetime booster of eIPV for school-age children

and adults who have completed a primary series of eIPV (OPV may also be used for this booster)

Contraindications

- An immediate anaphylactic reaction to a previous dose of eIPV vaccine
- Allergy to a vaccine component
  - History of anaphylactic reaction to streptomycin, polymyxin B, or neomycin
- Moderate or severe illnesses with or without a fever

Not Contraindications

- Pregnancy[1] or breast-feeding

Administration

- *Children:* 0.5 mL (unit dose) subcutaneously over the deltoid region (see page 67 for schedules)
- *Adults:*
  - Primary series: 3 0.5-mL doses subcutaneously over the deltoid region at 0, 1–2 months, and 6–12 months
  - If ≥8 weeks are available before protection is needed, 3 doses of IPV should be administered at least 4 weeks apart
  - If <8 weeks but >4 weeks are available before protection is needed, 2 doses of IPV should be administered at least 4 weeks apart
  - If <4 weeks are available before protection is needed, a single dose of OPV or IPV is recommended
  - Booster: a once-per-lifetime booster (OPV may also be used for persons who have received OPV or IPV previously) for adolescents and adults at future risk of exposure to poliomyelitis (e.g., international travel)

[1]It is prudent on theoretical grounds to avoid vaccinating pregnant women. However, if immediate protection against poliomyelitis is needed, OPV is preferred, although IPV may be considered if full vaccination can be completed before the anticipated imminent exposure.

ORAL POLIOVIRUS VACCINE (OPV)

Routine Indications

Routine use

- *Children:* universal immunization of children beginning at 6–8 weeks of age, using either the sequential IPV/OPV schedule or the OPV-only schedule (page 67)
- *Adolescents and adults:* (Adults ≥18 years of age living in the United States who never received or completed a primary series of polio vaccine do not need to be vaccinated unless otherwise indicated.)
  - A once-per-lifetime booster for persons who have completed a primary series of OPV or IPV (IPV may also be used for this booster) who are at increased risk for exposure to poliovirus: laboratory workers who handle specimens that may contain polioviruses and health-care workers directly providing care to patients who may be excreting poliovirus

International travel

- Travelers to areas or countries where poliomyelitis is epidemic or endemic
- IPV, OPV, or sequential IPV/OPV for children
- IPV for unimmunized or partially immunized adults
- A once-per-lifetime booster for persons who have completed a primary series of OPV or IPV (IPV may also be used for this booster) who are at increased risk for exposure to poliovirus

Contraindications

- An immediate anaphylactic reaction to a previous dose of OPV vaccine
- Moderate or severe acute illnesses with or without a fever
- Known immunodeficiency or altered immune status
  - Hematological and solid tumors
  - Congenital immunodeficiency
  - Long-term immunosuppressive therapy
  - HIV infection

  - A household contact who has an immunodeficiency or altered immune status (including HIV infection)
- An adult household contact known to be unvaccinated or inadequately vaccinated against poliomyelitis

Precautions[1]

- Recipients should avoid close contact with immunodeficient or immunocompromised individuals for at least 6–8 weeks following administration. If this is not feasible, rigorous hygiene and hand washing after contact with feces (e.g., after diaper changing) and avoidance of contact with saliva (e.g., sharing food or utensils) may be an acceptable but probably a less effective alternative.

Not Contraindications

- Pregnancy[2] or breast-feeding
- Current antimicrobial therapy
- Mild, acute illness with low-grade fever or mild diarrheal illness affecting an otherwise healthy child

Administration

- *Children:* 0.5 mL (unit dose) orally (see page 67 for schedules)
- *Adults:*
  - Primary series: not recommended (use IPV; page 63)
  - Booster: a once-per-lifetime booster (IPV may also be used) for adolescents and adults who have received 1 or more doses of OPV or IVP who are at future risk of exposure to poliomyelitis (e.g., international travel)
- The color of the vaccine before use (red, pink, or yellow) has no effect on the vaccine or efficacy

[1]No data exist to substantiate the theoretical risk of a suboptimal immune response from the administration of OPV and MMR within 30 days of each other.

[2]It is prudent on theoretical grounds to avoid vaccinating pregnant women. However, if immediate protection against poliomyelitis is needed, OPV is preferred, although eIPV may be considered if full vaccination can be completed before the anticipated imminent exposure.

- If a substantial amount of OPV is vomited or regurgitated within 5–10 minutes of administration, the dose should be administered again; if the repeat dose is not retained, neither dose should be counted and the vaccine should be readministered at a later visit

Poliovirus Vaccination Schedules for Children

	Child's Age			
Vaccination Schedule	**2 Months**	**4 Months**	**6–18 Months[1]**	**4–6 Years**
Recommended Schedule				
Sequential IVP/OPV	IPV	IPV	OPV	OPV
Alternative Schedules				
OPV only	OPV	OPV	OPV[1]	OPV
IPV only	IPV	IPV	IPV	IPV

[1]The ACIP recommends 2 doses of IPV at 2 and 4 months of age followed by 2 doses of OPV at 12–18 months and 4–6 years of age. The AAP and AAFP give no preference for any of the three acceptable schedules and recommend that, for children who received IPV at ages 2 and 4 months, the third dose of polio vaccine (either IPV or OPV) be administered at 6–18 months of age. IPV is the only poliovirus vaccine recommended for immunocompromised persons and their household contacts.

Comparison of Poliovirus Vaccines and Schedules

Characteristic	Killed (eIPV) Vaccine (Salk)	Live (OPV) Vaccine (Sabin)	Sequential eIPV-OPV Schedule
Efficacy			
Number of serotypes in vaccine	3	3	3
Prevents paralytic polio	Yes	Yes	Yes
Administration route	Subcutaneous	Oral	Subcutaneous and oral
Number of doses in primary series	3	3	3
Booster at 4–6 years	Yes	Yes	Yes
Immunity			
Induces systemic humoral immunity	High	High	High
Induces mucosal immunity in the gastrointestinal tract	Low	High	High
Gastrointestinal tract reinfection	Yes	Brief	Unknown
Duration of immunity	Uncertain; probably lifelong	Lifelong	Uncertain; probably lifelong
Adverse Events			
Virus excretion of vaccine virus	None	1–3 weeks	Some
Occurrence of vaccine-associated paralytic poliomyelitis (VAPP)	None	8–9 cases/year	2–5 cases/year *(estimated)*
Other serious adverse events	None	None	None
Additional Issues			
Cost	High	Low	Intermediate
Extra injections or visits required	Yes	No	Yes
Expected compliance	Possibly reduced	High	Possibly reduced
Future combination vaccines	Likely	Unlikely	Likely with eIPV

Rotavirus Vaccine[1]

Routine Indications

Routine use

- Universal immunization of all infants beginning at 2 months of age[1] (the first dose should be given by 6 months of age)

International travel

- All infants should be immunized routinely

Contraindications

- Persistent vomiting or diarrhea
- Moderate or severe acute illness with or without a fever may be a contraindication depending on the etiology and the physician's assessment
- Altered immunocompetence
  - Hematological and solid tumors
  - Congenital immunodeficiency (including agammaglobulinemia)
  - Long-term immunosuppressive therapy
  - HIV infection (including asymptomatic HIV-seropositive infants)

Precautions

- The vaccine may be used in premature (<37 weeks' gestation) infants but the safety and efficacy in premature infants are not established

Not Contraindications

- Pregnancy (in a hospital contact) or breast-feeding

---

[1]The ACIP made a preliminary recommendation in February 1998 for routine use of the rotavirus vaccine. Rotavirus vaccine received FDA approval on August 31, 1998. Final ACIP/CDC, AAP, and AAFP recommendations are pending as of September 1, 1998. For updated information, see www.vaccine.uthscsa.edu.

Administration

- Lyophilized vaccine is reconstituted with 2.5 mL of citrate-bicarbonate diluent immediately before administration of 2.5 mL orally, administered at 2, 4, and 6 months of age (at least 3 weeks apart)
- Administer reconstituted vaccine within 30 minutes

Varicella (Chickenpox) Vaccine

Routine Indications

Routine use

- Children 12–18 months of age
- Children 19 months through 12 years of age who have not been previously immunized and who lack a reliable history of chickenpox

High-risk groups

- Susceptible household contacts of immunocompromised individuals
- All health-care workers[1] (page 24)

International travel

- All children through 12 years of age should be immunized routinely
- Adult international travelers who are known to be susceptible to varicella

Possible Indications

- Individuals who live or work in environments with a high likelihood of transmission of varicella-zoster virus (VZV):
  - Teachers of young children
  - Employees of child day care centers
  - Residents and staff in institutional settings
- Individuals who live or work in environments in which VZV transmission may occur:
  - College students
  - Inmates and staff of correctional institutions
  - Military personnel
- Nonpregnant women of childbearing age

[1]All health-care workers (i.e., medical or nonmedical, paid or volunteer, full-time or part-time, student or nonstudent, with or without patient-care responsibilities) who work in facilities that provide health care to patients (i.e., inpatient or outpatient, public or private) should be immune to measles, rubella, and varicella.

Contraindications

- An immediate anaphylactic reaction to a previous dose of VZV vaccine
- Allergy to a vaccine component
  - History of anaphylactic reaction to neomycin or gelatin
- Moderate or severe illnesses with or without a fever
- Varicella or herpes zoster within the previous 21 days
- Pregnancy, women should be counseled to avoid pregnancy for 1 month after administration of varicella vaccine
- Active untreated tuberculosis
- Immunocompromised individuals, including the following:
  - Persons with leukemia, lymphoma, or other malignancies
  - Persons receiving radiotherapy or chemotherapy
  - HIV-infected individuals
  - Persons taking high-dose corticosteroids (≥2 mg/kg/day of prednisone, or equivalent, for more than 1 month until 1–3 months after discontinuing corticosteroids)

Precautions

- Women should be counseled to avoid pregnancy for 1 month after administration of varicella vaccine
- Recent immune globulin administration[2] (page 112)
- Immune globulin products should not be administered for at least 3 weeks after vaccination
- If MMR vaccine is not given at the same time, MMR and varicella vaccine should be administered at least 30 days apart
- Salicylates should be avoided for 6 weeks after receiving varicella vaccine (to minimize the theoretical risk of Reye syndrome)
- Persons with a family history of primary immunodeficiency should be evaluated for immune competence before varicella vaccination

---

[2]If an immune globulin is administered in the interval before vaccination is recommended (page 112), the recipient should be revaccinated at or after the appropriate interval unless serological testing indicates that varicella-specific antibodies were induced.

- Vaccine recipients should avoid, whenever possible, close contact with high-risk susceptible individuals for 6 weeks after vaccination

Special Considerations

- Unreconstituted (lyophilized) vaccine storage
  - Must be stored at an average temperature of −15°C (5°F) or colder
  - May be stored in a container with dry ice for shipping or temporary storage to maintain these temperatures
  - May be stored in a refrigerator at 3.3°C (38°F) for up to 72 hours, after which it must be discarded
- Reconstituted vaccine storage
  - Must be used within 30 minutes, after which it must be discarded

Not Contraindications

- Immunocompromised household member
- Pregnancy of the mother (or another household member) of the recipient
- Breast-feeding

Administration

- 0.5 mL subcutaneously in the deltoid region

Schedule for Routine Administration

Age	Dose (plaque-forming units [PFU])	Volume (mL)	Number of Doses	Schedule
12 months to 13 years	≥1500	0.5	1	1 dose
≥13 years	≥1500	0.5	2	4–8 weeks apart

Combination Vaccines for Routine Immunizations of Children

TETRAMUNE

- Combines HibTITER (*H. influenzae* type b conjugate [HbOC], 10 μg) and Tri-Immunol (DTwP) vaccines

Administration

- Administered intramuscularly at 2, 4, 6, and 12–15 months (constitutes the Hib and DTP primary series and the boosters)

TriHIBit

- Combines ActHIB (*H. influenzae* type b conjugate vaccine [PRP-T] 10 μg) by reconstitution with Tripedia (DTaP vaccine produced by Pasteur Mérieux Connaught)

Administration

- Administered intramuscularly at 15–18 months (constitutes the Hib and DTP boosters)

COMVAX

- Combines PedvaxHIB (*H. influenzae* type b conjugate [PRP-OMP], 7.5 μg) and Recombivax HB (hepatitis B, 5 μg) vaccines
- Infants born to HBsAg-positive mothers should receive hepatitis B immune globulin (HBIG) and the first dose of hepatitis B vaccine (Engerix-B or Recombivax HB, not Comvax) at birth (page 205)
- Infants born to mothers of unknown HBsAg status should receive hepatitis B vaccine (Engerix-B or Recombivax HB, not Comvax) at birth (page 205)

Administration

- Administered intramuscularly at 2, 4, and 12–15 months (constitutes the Hib and HB primary series)
- Comvax should not be administered to infants <6 weeks of age

- Comvax may be administered to infants given 1 dosc of hepatitis B at or shortly after birth

Schedules Incorporating Comvax

Birth	2 Months	4 Months	12–15 Months
Hepatitis B #1	Comvax	PedvaxHIB	Comvax
or			
Hepatitis B #1	Comvax	Comvax	Comvax

FREQUENTLY USED SPECIAL VACCINES

Hepatitis A Vaccine

Routine Indications

Routine use

- Not recommended for universal use

High-risk groups[1]

- Children ≥2 years of age in communities with high endemic rates (peak rates of ≥700 cases per 100,000 population) or periodic outbreaks
  - Alaskan natives
  - Native Americans
  - Pacific Islanders
  - Selected Hispanic communities (e.g., border regions with Mexico)
  - Selected religious communities (e.g., Hasidic Jews)
- Male homosexuals
- Users of illegal drugs
- Persons with chronic liver disease, including those who are awaiting or who have received liver transplants
- Hemophiliac patients and other recipients of certain blood products (clotting-factor concentrates)
- Food handlers where local health authorities or private employers determine vaccination to be cost effective
- Persons who have occupational risk for infection
  - Persons who work with hepatitis A–infected primates or hepatitis A virus in a research laboratory setting
- Health-care workers (page 24)
  - Routine preexposure prophylaxis (vaccination) of all health-care workers is not recommended

[1]Prevaccination screening is likely to be cost effective for hepatitis A for persons >40 years of age as well as for younger persons in certain groups with a high prevalence of hepatitis A infection.

  - In documented outbreaks of hepatitis A infection, IG postexposure prophylaxis is recommended for health-care workers who are exposed to feces of infected patients and who do not use proper precautions

Outbreak control

- In communities with high rates of hepatitis A and periodic outbreaks (peak rates of ≥700 reported cases per 100,000 population), routine vaccination of children ≥2 years of age and catch-up vaccination of older children are recommended
- In communities with intermediate rates of hepatitis A (50–200 reported cases per 100,000 population), vaccination programs targeting subpopulations with the highest rates of disease may be considered

International travel

- International travelers ≥2 years of age to countries with intermediate or high hepatitis A endemicity (countries other than the United States, Canada, Australia, New Zealand, Japan, western Europe, and Scandinavia)

Possible Indications

High-risk groups

- Individuals ≥2 years of age who live or work in environments in which hepatitis A transmission may occur[2]
  - Military personnel
  - Caretakers of developmentally challenged persons
  - Food handlers
  - Staff of child day care centers

International travel

- Travelers ≥2 years of age to developed areas of the Caribbean

Postexposure prophylaxis

- In combination with immune globulin (IG) for individuals requiring both immediate and short-term protection (page 164)

---

[2]Health-care workers, food handlers, teachers of young children, day care center staff, and sewage workers (in the United States) have not been shown to be at increased risk of hepatitis A infection because of occupational exposure.

Contraindications

- An immediate anaphylactic reaction to a previous dose of any hepatitis A vaccine
  - Allergy to a vaccine component
  - History of hypersensitivity reactions to alum or, in the case of Havrix, to the preservative 2-phenoxyethanol
- Moderate or severe illnesses with or without a fever

Not Contraindications

- Immunocompromised persons
- Pregnancy (The safety in pregnancy has not been determined although the theoretical risk is low.)

Administration[1]

Age (Years)	Dose	Volume (mL)	Number of Doses	Schedule[2] (Months)
Havrix (SmithKline Beecham)				
2–18	720 EL.U.	0.5	2	0, 6–12
>18	1440 EL.U.	1	2	0, 6–12
Vaqta (Merck)				
2–17	25 units	0.5	2	0, 6–18
≥18	50 units	1	2	0, 6

EL.U. = enzyme-linked immunosorbent assay units.

[1]Administration by intramuscular injection into the deltoid muscle.

[2]0 months represents the time of the first dose; subsequent doses are given in the recommended intervals after the first dose.

Influenza Vaccine

Routine Indications

Routine use

- Not recommended for universal use in children
- Individuals ≥65 years of age
- Anyone who desires to reduce the likelihood of becoming ill with influenza

High-risk groups for severe influenza or complications

- Individuals ≥65 years of age
- Residents of nursing homes and other chronic-care facilities that house persons of any age who have chronic medical conditions
- Adults and children with a chronic cardiovascular disorder (hemodynamically significant cardiac disease)
- Adults and children with a chronic pulmonary disorder, including children with asthma
- Adults and children who required regular medical follow-up or hospitalization during the preceding year because of the following:
  - Diabetes
  - Other chronic metabolic diseases
  - Renal dysfunction
  - Hemoglobinopathies
  - Immunosuppression (including immunosuppression caused by medications, and persons with HIV infection)
- Children and adolescents (6 months of age to 18 years of age) receiving long-term aspirin therapy (i.e., for rheumatoid arthritis or Kawasaki syndrome) and who therefore might be at risk of developing Reye syndrome after influenza
- Women who will be in the second or third trimester (≥14 weeks' gestation) of pregnancy during the influenza season (December through March)[1]

---

[1]Influenza infection may cause increased morbidity in women during the second and third trimesters of pregnancy. Women who will be beyond the first trimester of pregnancy (≥14 weeks' gestation) during the influenza season should be vaccinated. Pregnant women who have medical conditions that increase their risk

- Persons, including health-care workers, who can transmit influenza to persons at high risk for complications
  - Household members (including children) of persons in high-risk groups
  - Physicians, nurses, and other health-care workers in hospital and outpatient-care settings
  - Health-care workers in nursing homes and chronic-care facilities who have contact with patients or residents
  - Providers of home health care (e.g., visiting nurses, volunteer workers) to persons at high risk

International travel

- All travelers should be vaccinated with influenza vaccine if otherwise indicated

Contraindications

- An immediate anaphylactic reaction to a previous dose of any influenza virus vaccine
- Allergy to a vaccine component
  - History of anaphylactic hypersensitivity (e.g., urticaria, swelling of the mouth and throat, difficulty breathing, hypotension, or shock) to eggs or egg proteins[2]
- Moderate or severe illnesses with or without a fever
- Age <6 months
- Persons with an active neurological disorder or a history of neurological symptoms or signs after influenza vaccination

---

for complications from influenza should be vaccinated before the influenza season, regardless of the stage of pregnancy. No adverse fetal effects have been associated with influenza vaccine. Because influenza vaccine is not a live-virus vaccine and major systemic reactions to it are rare, many experts consider influenza vaccination safe during any stage of pregnancy. However, because spontaneous abortion is common in the first trimester and unnecessary exposures have traditionally been avoided during this time, some experts prefer influenza vaccination during the second trimester to avoid coincidental association of the vaccine with early pregnancy loss.

[2]Persons with a history of anaphylactic reactions following egg ingestion should be vaccinated with caution (page 114). Use of antiviral agent (amantadine or rimantadine) is an option for prevention of influenza A in such persons (page 175).

- Persons with a history of Guillain-Barré syndrome (stated as a contraindication by the FDA and the manufacturer, but not by the ACIP)

Not Contraindications

- Pregnancy or breast-feeding
- Minor illnesses (e.g., upper respiratory tract infection, allergic rhinitis) with or without a fever

Administration[1]

- Optimal time for immunization is from October 1 through mid-November, but any time from September to the end of the influenza season (as long as cases are still occurring) is appropriate

Age	Product[2]	Dosage	Number of Doses
6–35 months	Split virus only[3]	0.25 mL	Initial series: 2 doses at least 1 month apart (with the second dose before December if possible); 1 dose annually thereafter
3–8 years	Split virus only[3]	0.5 mL	Initial series: 2 doses at least 1 month apart (with the second dose before December if possible); 1 dose annually thereafter
9–12 years	Split virus only[3]	0.5 mL	1 dose (initially and annually)
≥12 years	Whole or split virus[3]	0.5 mL	1 dose (initially and annually)

Adapted from Centers for Disease Control and Prevention. Prevention and control of influenza. Recommendations of the Advisory Committee on Immunization Practices (ACIP). *MMWR Morb Mortal Wkly Rep* 1998;47 (RR-6):5.

[1]Administration by intramuscular injection into the deltoid muscle (or anterolateral mid-thigh for children <24 months of age).

[2]Manufacturers include Connaught Laboratories (Fluzone whole or split); Evans Medical/Medeva Pharmaceuticals (Fluvirin purified surface antigen vaccine), and Wyeth-Ayerst Laboratories (FluShield split).

[3]Because of their decreased potential for causing febrile reactions, only split-virus vaccines should be used in children. They may be labeled as "split," "subvirion," or "purified surface antigen" vaccine. Immunogenicity and side effects of split- and whole-virus vaccines are similar among adults when vaccines are administered at the recommended dosage.

Meningococcus (*Neisseria meningitidis*) Vaccine

Routine Indications

Routine use

- Not recommended for universal use

High-risk groups (≥2 years of age)

- Functional or anatomical asplenia
- Deficiency of a terminal component of complement (C5–C9)
- Properdin deficiency
- Military recruits
- Target groups identified by local/state public health authorities during an outbreak or cluster of cases caused by a vaccine-preventable serogroup (A, C, Y, W-135)
- Routine preexposure prophylaxis (vaccination) of all health-care workers is not recommended

International travel

- Patients ≥2 years of age traveling to or residing in a country with hyperendemic or epidemic meningococcal disease caused by a vaccine-preventable serogroup (A, C, Y, W-135)
- Infants ≥3 months of age traveling to an area with hyperendemic or epidemic serogroup A meningococcal disease

Contraindications

- An immediate anaphylactic reaction to a previous dose of meningococcus vaccine
- Allergy to a vaccine component
  - Anaphylactic reaction to thimerosal
- Moderate or severe illnesses with or without a fever

Not Contraindications

- Pregnancy or breast-feeding

Administration

- 0.5 mL as a single dose subcutaneously or by jet injection

Pneumococcus (*Streptococcus pneumoniae*) Vaccine[1]

Routine Indications

Routine use

- Not recommended for universal use in children
- Individuals ≥65 years of age
- Persons who received the 14-valent pneumococcus vaccine (distributed from 1987–1983)
- Revaccination of persons ≥65 years of age who received vaccine ≥5 years previously and were <65 years of age at the time of vaccination
- Revaccination of persons 2–64 years of age with functional or anatomical asplenia or who are immunocompromised

High-risk groups (≥2 years of age)

- Persons with functional or anatomical asplenia (including sickle cell disease and splenectomy)[2]
- Persons with chronic illness at increased risk

Strong epidemiological evidence and substantial clinical benefit support vaccine use

- Chronic cardiovascular disease (including congestive heart failure and cardiomyopathies)
- Chronic pulmonary disease (including chronic obstructive pulmonary disease and emphysema, but not asthma)
- Diabetes mellitus

Moderate evidence supports vaccine use

- Alcoholism
- Chronic liver disease (including cirrhosis)
- Cerebrospinal fluid leaks

---

[1]Pneumococcus vaccines include purified polysaccharide antigens of 23 serotypes (U.S. nomenclature: 1, 2, 3, 4, 5, 8, 9, 12, 13, 17, 19, 20, 22, 23, 26, 34, 43, 51, 56, 57, 68, 70; Danish nomenclature: 1, 2, 3, 4, 5, 6B, 7F, 8, 9N, 9V, 10A, 11A, 12F, 14, 15B, 17F, 18C, 19A, 19F, 20, 22F, 23F, 33F). These 23 types represent at least 85%–90% of the >80 serotypes that cause invasive pneumococcal infection in the United States and include the six serotypes (6B, 9V, 14, 19A, 19F, and 23F) that most frequently cause invasive drug-resistant pneumococcal infection in the United States.

[2]These individuals should be considered for revaccination.

Effectiveness is not proven, but high risk supports vaccine use

- Immunocompromised persons[2]:
  - HIV infection, leukemia, lymphoma, Hodgkin disease, multiple myeloma, generalized malignancy[2]
  - Chronic renal failure or nephrotic syndrome[2]
  - Receiving immunosuppressive chemotherapy, including corticosteroids[2]
  - Organ or bone marrow transplant[2]
- Persons living in special environments or social settings who are at increased risk:
  - Alaskan natives and certain American Indian populations
  - Residents of nursing homes or long-term care facilities
  - Military recruits
- Routine preexposure prophylaxis (vaccination) of all health-care workers is not recommended

International travel

- All travelers should be vaccinated with pneumococcus vaccine if otherwise indicated

Contraindications

- An immediate anaphylactic reaction to a previous dose of pneumococcus vaccine
- Allergy to a vaccine component:
  - Anaphylactic reaction to phenol or thimerosal
- Moderate or severe illnesses with or without a fever

Not Contraindications

- Pregnancy or breast-feeding

Administration

- 0.5 mL subcutaneously or intramuscularly, preferably in the deltoid muscle (or anterolateral mid-thigh for children <24 months of age)

Booster dose[3]

- Persons ≥65 years of age who received vaccine ≥5 years previously and were <65 years of age at the time of vaccination
- Persons 2–64 years of age with the following:
  - Functional or anatomical asplenia (including sickle cell disease and splenectomy)
  - HIV infection, leukemia, lymphoma, Hodgkin disease, multiple myeloma, generalized malignancy
  - Chronic renal failure or nephrotic syndrome
  - Receiving immunosuppressive chemotherapy, including corticosteroids
  - Organ or bone marrow transplant

Timing

- If ≤10 years of age at revaccination, consider a single revaccination 3 years after first dose
- If >10 years of age at revaccination, a single revaccination ≥5 years after first dose

Administration

- Same as for initial dose

[3]Revaccination following a second dose is not routinely recommended.

Rabies Vaccine

Routine Indications

Routine use

- Postexposure prophylaxis for rabies for certain wounds (page 183)
- Preexposure immunization of persons with risk of exposure to rabies

Risk Category	Nature of Risk	Typical Populations	Preexposure Recommendations
Continuous	Virus present continuously, often in high concentrations Aerosol, mucous membrane, bite, or nonbite exposure Specific exposures may go unrecognized	Rabies research laboratory workers; rabies biological production workers	Primary course Serological testing every 6 months Booster vaccination when antibody level falls below acceptable level[1]
Frequent	Exposure usually episodic, with source recognized, but exposure may also be unrecognized Aerosol, mucous membrane, bite, or nonbite exposure	Rabies diagnostic laboratory workers, spelunkers, veterinarians and staff, and animal-control and wildlife workers in rabies enzootic areas Travelers visiting foreign areas of enzootic rabies for >30 days	Primary course Serological testing or booster vaccination every 2 years[1]

[1]Minimum acceptable antibody level is complete virus neutralization at a 1:5 serum dilution by rapid fluorescent focus inhibition test (RFFIT). This dilution is approximately equal to the minimum titer of 0.5 IU recommended by WHO. Booster dose should be administered if the titer falls below this level.

Risk Category	Nature of Risk	Typical Populations	Preexposure Recommendations
Infrequent (greater than the population at large)	Exposure nearly always episodic with source recognized Mucous membrane, bite, or nonbite exposure	Veterinarians and animal-control and wildlife workers in areas of low rabies enzooticity, veterinary students	Primary course No serological testing or booster vaccination
Rare (population at large)	Exposure always episodic Mucous membrane, or bite with source unrecognized	U.S. population at large, including persons in rabies enzootic areas	No preexposure vaccination necessary

Adapted from Centers for Disease Control and Prevention. Rabies Prevention–United States, 1991. Recommendations of the Immunization Practices Advisory Committee (ACIP). *MMWR Morb Mortal Wkly Rep* 1991;40 (RR-3):1–19.

International travel

- Travelers living in or visiting areas of endemic dog rabies (most countries in Central and South America, the Indian subcontinent, Southeast Asia [except Japan and Taiwan], and most of Africa) for >30 days
- Travelers to developing countries whose occupation or activities place them at frequent risk of exposure (e.g., hunters, forest rangers, taxidermists, laboratory workers, stock breeders, slaughterhouse workers, veterinarians, spelunkers)
- If chloroquine or mefloquine is administered for malaria prophylaxis, the intramuscular vaccine should be used

Precaution

- Human diploid cell vaccine (HDCV) should not be administered by the intradermal route if chloroquine, mefloquine, or other structurally related antimalarial agents are administered

Contraindications

- An immediate anaphylactic reaction to a previous dose of rabies vaccine
- Allergy to a vaccine component

Not Contraindications

- Pregnancy or breast-feeding
- Allergy to a vaccine component: the risks of vaccination must be weighed against the risk of rabies. Consultation with an expert is recommended for persons thought to have an allergy to rabies vaccine

Administration

Age	Volume (mL)	Number of Doses	Schedule
HDCV (Imovax Rabies), PCEC (RabAvert), or RVA[1]			
Primary series	1	3	0, 7, and 21 or 28 days
Booster	1		1 dose
HDCV (Imovax Rabies I.D.)[2]			
Primary series	0.1	3	0, 7, and 21 or 28 days
Booster	0.1		1 dose

[1]Administration is by intramuscular injection in the deltoid muscle. The deltoid area is the only acceptable site of vaccination for adults and older children. For children <24 months of age, the anterolateral aspect of the mid-thigh may be used. HDCV should never be administered in the gluteal region.

[2]If chloroquine, mefloquine, or other structurally related antimalarial agents are administered for malaria prophylaxis, the intramuscular vaccine should be used.

Typhoid Fever *(Salmonella typhi)* Vaccine

Routine Indications

Routine use

- Not recommended for universal use

High-risk groups (≥2 years of age)

- Household contacts of documented *S. typhi* carriers
- Sewage sanitation workers in typhoid endemic areas (outside the United States)
- Workers in microbiology laboratories who frequently work with *S. typhi* (Vaccination is not an alternative to the use of proper procedures when handling specimens and cultures in the laboratory.)
- Routine preexposure prophylaxis (vaccination) of all health-care workers is not recommended

International travel

- Travelers to endemic areas of developing countries (especially Africa, Asia, and South and Central America), especially if prolonged exposure to potentially contaminated food and water is likely; the vaccine regimen should be completed at least 2 weeks (parenteral purified polysaccharide or inactivated whole-cell vaccines) or 1 week (oral live-attenuated strain of *S. typhi* strain Ty21a) before potential exposure

Precautions

- If malaria prophylaxis with mefloquine is also to be provided, the oral Ty21a vaccine should not be administered 24 hours before or after a dose of mefloquine

Contraindications

- An immediate anaphylactic reaction to a previous dose of vaccine
- Allergy to a vaccine component
- Moderate or severe illnesses with or without a fever
- *For oral live-attenuated typhoid vaccine only:*
  - Persons with an acute febrile illness or acute gastrointestinal illness
  - Persons taking antibiotics

  - Immunocompromised individuals
  - HIV-infected persons

Not Contraindications

- Pregnancy or breast-feeding

Administration: Comparison of Vaccines for Typhoid Fever (Salmonella typhi)

	Vi Capsular Polysaccharide Vaccine	Heat-phenol Inactivated Vaccine	Oral Live-attenuated Vaccine (Ty21a)
Type of vaccine	Purified polysaccharide antigen (strain Ty2)	Inactivated whole-cell (strain Ty2)	Live-attenuated *S. typhi* strain Ty21a (2–6 × 10^9 CFU of viable *S. typhi* organisms per capsule, plus 5-50 × 10^9 nonviable bacterial cells)
Recommended age	≥2 years	≥6 months	≥6 years
Administration	Intramuscular[1]	Subcutaneous	Oral[2]
Primary vaccination	Single 0.5-mL injection	2 injections 4 weeks apart: 6 months–10 years: 0.25 mL ≥10 years: 0.5 mL	4 oral doses on alternate days
Booster	Every 2 years (0.5 mL)	Every 3 years *Subcutaneous:* <10 years: 0.25 mL ≥10 years: 0.5 mL *Intradermal:* ≥6 months: 0.1 mL	Every 5 years (4 oral doses on alternate days)
Adverse reactions			
Fever	0%–1%	7%–24%	0%–5%
Headache	1%–3%	9%–10%	0%–5%
Local reactions	7% (erythema or induration ≥1 cm)	3%–35% (severe local pain or swelling)	Rare abdominal discomfort, nausea, vomiting, rash, or urticaria

[1]Administration is by intramuscular injection in the deltoid muscle. For children <24 months of age, the anterolateral aspect of the mid-thigh may be used. Do not administer in the gluteal region.

[2]The oral vaccine should be swallowed with a cold or lukewarm drink on an empty stomach approximately 1 hour before eating. The capsules should be stored in a refrigerator until taken. The capsules should not be opened and should not be taken with alcohol.

INFREQUENTLY USED SPECIAL VACCINES

Bacille Calmette-Guérin (BCG) Vaccine

Routine Indications

Routine use

- Not recommended for universal use

High-risk groups

- Children who are continuously exposed to an untreated or ineffectively treated person with infectious pulmonary tuberculosis if the child cannot be removed from the environment
- Children who are continuously exposed to an individual with multidrug-resistant tuberculosis if the child cannot be removed from the environment
- Health-care workers in areas where multidrug tuberculosis is prevalent, a strong likelihood of exposure exists, and comprehensive infection control precautions have been implemented but have failed to prevent tuberculosis transmission to health-care workers; vaccination with BCG should not be routinely recommended or required for employment or assignment in specific work areas

International travel

- Not currently recommended or required for international travel

Possible Indications

- Intravesical instillation for prophylaxis against recurrent papillary carcinoma of the urinary bladder

Contraindications

- An immediate anaphylactic reaction to a previous dose of vaccine
- Allergy to a vaccine component
- Moderate or severe illnesses with or without a fever
- Altered immunocompetence
  - Hematological and solid tumors
  - Congenital immunodeficiency

  - Long-term immunosuppressive therapy
  - Infection with HIV
- Pregnancy
- As a requirement of employment of health-care workers
- For health-care workers employed in settings where the risk of transmission is low

Administration

- By percutaneous multiple-puncture disk. A volume of 0.2–0.3 mL (children <1 month of age receive one half the dose by diluting the vaccine) of vaccine is placed onto cleansed skin, a sterile multiple-puncture (36-point) disk is used for percutaneous penetration of tensed skin, the disk is rocked forward and backward and from side to side several times, the disk is removed, and vaccine is spread evenly over the puncture sites with the wide edge of the disk and allowed to dry. No dressing is required. The site should be kept dry for 24 hours. A normal reaction consists of small red papules appearing at 10–14 days that may reach a maximum diameter of 3 mm after 4–6 weeks, after which they may scale and slowly subside. A round scar may persist permanently. The anatomical site of vaccination is not standardized, but the upper arm is preferred.
- Persons who remain negative to a 5-TU tuberculin skin test after 2–3 months should have a repeat vaccination. Infants who remain negative to a 5-TU tuberculin skin test, and if indications for BCG vaccination persist, should receive a full BCG dose after 1 year of age.
- Routine booster doses are not recommended.

Cholera (*Vibrio cholerae*) Vaccine

Routine Indications

Routine use

- Not recommended for universal use

International travel

- Persons traveling to areas where local authorities require cholera vaccination
  - **Currently no country or territory requires cholera vaccination as a condition for entry. Local authorities, however, may continue to require documentation of cholera vaccination; in such cases, a single dose of vaccine is sufficient to satisfy local requirements. Persons following the usual tourist itinerary who use standard accommodations in countries reporting cholera are at virtually no risk of infection.**
- No country requires proof of cholera vaccination as a condition for entry, and the International Certificate of Vaccination no longer provides a specific space for recording cholera vaccination
- Cholera vaccine induces incomplete, unreliable protection of short duration, and its use therefore is not recommended; cholera vaccine is only approximately 50% effective in reducing clinical illness, with the greatest protection during the first 2 months following immunization, and does not protect against non-O1 serotypes of cholera, such as *V. cholerae* O139
- Travelers to cholera-infected areas should take appropriate food precautions (page 270)
- Vaccination against cholera cannot prevent the introduction of the infection into a country; the World Health Assembly therefore amended the International Health Regulations in 1973 so that cholera vaccination is no longer required of any traveler

Contraindications

- An immediate anaphylactic reaction to a previous dose of vaccine

- Allergy to a vaccine component
- Moderate or severe illnesses with or without a fever
- Age <6 months (no data are available on the safety and efficacy)
- Pregnancy (may be administered if required for local travel)
- Concurrent cholera and yellow fever vaccination impairs the immune response to each vaccine; these vaccines should be administered at a minimal interval of 3 weeks unless precluded by time constraints, when they should be given on the same day

Administration

	Subcutaneous or Intramuscular Injection			Intradermal[1]	
Regimen	**6 Months–4 Years**	**5–10 Years**	**>10 Years**	**≥5 Years**	**Schedule**
Primary series	0.2 mL	0.3 mL	0.5 mL	0.2 mL	2 doses given 1 week to ≥1 month apart
Booster[2]	0.2 mL	0.3 mL	0.5 mL	0.2 mL	1 dose every 6 months

[1]Do not administer intradermally in children <5 years of age.
[2]Maximize protection by giving the booster dose at the beginning of the season.

Japanese Encephalitis Vaccine

Routine Indications

Routine use

- Laboratory workers with a potential for exposure to infectious Japanese encephalitis virus

International travel[1]

- Persons traveling for ≥1 month in endemic areas (People's Republic of China, Korea, the Indian subcontinent [India, parts of Bangladesh, southern Nepal, Sri Lanka], Southeast Asia [Burma, Thailand, Cambodia, Laos, Vietnam, Malaysia, Indonesia, the Philippines], with lower frequency in Japan, Taiwan, Singapore, Hong Kong, and eastern Russia) during the transmission season (May to September in temperate climates; variable in subtropical and tropical areas with rainfall, the rainy season, and the migratory patterns of avian-amplifying hosts) if travel will include rural areas
- Persons traveling for <30 days in areas experiencing epidemic transmission

Possible Indications

- Persons traveling for <30 days in endemic areas whose activities (e.g., extensive outdoor activities in rural areas) place them at high risk for exposure
- Persons >55 years of age may be at higher risk for disease after infection and should be carefully considered for vaccination if they travel in areas of risk

Contraindications

- An immediate anaphylactic reaction to a previous dose of vaccine
- Allergy to a vaccine component
  - History of anaphylactic hypersensitivity (e.g., urticaria, swelling of the mouth and throat, difficulty breathing, hypotension, or shock) to eggs or egg proteins

---

[1]All travelers to these areas are advised to use precautions to avoid mosquito bites (page 269).

- Moderate or severe illnesses with or without a fever
- Pregnancy (Pregnant women who must travel to an area where the risk of Japanese encephalitis is high should be vaccinated when the theoretical risks of immunization are outweighed by the risk of infection to the mother and developing fetus.)
- Immunocompromised persons
- Age <1 year (No data are available on the safety and efficacy; whenever possible vaccination should be deferred until age ≥1 year.)

Administration[1]

Age	Volume (mL)	Number of Doses	Schedule
1–3 Years			
Primary series[2]	0.5	3	0, 7, and 30 days
Booster	0.5	1	Every 2 years
≥3 Years			
Primary series[2]	1	3	0, 7, and 30 days
Booster	1	1	Every 2 years

[1]The last dose should be administered at least 10 days before the commencement of travel.

[2]An abbreviated but less effective schedule of 0, 7, and 14 days can be used when the recommended schedule is impractical or inconvenient because of time constraints. Two doses administered 1 week apart will confer short-term immunity in 80% of vaccinees, although this schedule is not recommended and should be used only under unusual circumstances.

Plague (*Yersinia pestis*) Vaccine

Routine Indications

Routine use

- Laboratory personnel 18–61 years of age who routinely perform procedures that involve *Y. pestis*
- Persons (e.g., mammalogists, ecologists, and other field workers) 18–61 years of age who have regular contact with wild rodents or their fleas in areas in which plague is enzootic or epizootic

International travel

- Not currently recommended or required for international travel

Contraindications

- An immediate anaphylactic reaction to a previous dose of vaccine
- Allergy to a vaccine component
- Moderate or severe illnesses with or without a fever
- Age ≤17 years or ≥62 years (insufficient data are available for these age-groups)
- Pregnancy (may use selectively in pregnancy for vaccination of exposed persons)[1]

Administration

- Three intramuscular injections, preferably in the deltoid muscle:
  - 1 mL
  - 0.2 mL 1–3 months after the first injection
  - 0.2 mL 5–6 months after the second injection
- Booster doses of 0.2 mL can be administered at 1- to 2-year intervals for individuals who remain at risk for infection, or at 6-month intervals for individuals who remain at high risk for infection

---

[1]Women should be asked if they are pregnant before vaccination and should be advised to avoid becoming pregnant for 1 month following each dose of vaccine.

Vaccinia (Smallpox) Vaccine

Routine Indications

Routine use

- Military recruits

High-risk groups

- Laboratory workers (primarily researchers) who directly handle cultures of vaccinia, recombinant vaccinia viruses, or orthopoxviruses
- May be considered for other health-care workers whose contact with orthopoxviruses is limited to contaminated dressings or other infectious materials
- Routine preexposure prophylaxis (vaccination) of all health-care workers is not recommended

International travel

- Smallpox vaccination is not required by any country

Possible Indications

- Health-care workers involved with contaminated materials from clinical trials using recombinant vaccinia viruses

Contraindications

- An immediate anaphylactic reaction to a previous dose of vaccine
- Allergy to a vaccine component
- Moderate or severe illnesses with or without a fever
- Persons with eczema or other exfoliative skin conditions, atopic dermatitis, impetigo, chickenpox, wounds, or burns, and household contacts of such persons because of an increased risk of eczema vaccinatum
- Immunosuppressed persons

Administration

- Percutaneous scarification using a bifurcated needle, traditionally at a site over the upper deltoid; a residual scar indicates prior vaccination
- Booster doses of 15 punctures at 10-year intervals

Yellow Fever Vaccine

Routine Indications

Routine use

- Not recommended for universal use

International travel[1]

- **Yellow fever is the *only* disease for which countries may require an International Certificate of Vaccination under WHO guidelines. Some countries require a yellow fever vaccination for all travelers, whereas others only require a vaccination if a traveler is coming *from* either areas infected with yellow fever or areas where yellow fever transmission has occurred (endemic areas)**
- Persons ≥9 months of age traveling to or living in areas of tropical South America and Africa where yellow fever infection is officially reported
- Persons ≥9 months of age traveling to or living in rural areas of countries that do not officially report the disease but that lie in the yellow fever endemic zone
- Infants <9 months of age and pregnant women should be considered for vaccination if traveling to areas experiencing ongoing epidemic yellow fever when travel cannot be postponed and a high level of protection against mosquito exposure is not feasible

Contraindications

- An immediate anaphylactic reaction to a previous dose of vaccine
- Allergy to a vaccine component
  - Persons with histories of anaphylactic hypersensitivity (e.g., urticaria, swelling of the mouth and throat, difficulty breathing, hypotension, or shock) to eggs or egg proteins[2]
- Moderate or severe illnesses with or without a fever

---

[1]All travelers to these areas are advised to use precautions to avoid mosquito bites (page 269).

[2]Persons with a history of anaphylactic reactions following egg ingestion should be vaccinated with caution (page 114).

- Age <1 year (No data are available on the safety and efficacy in children. Whenever possible, vaccination should be deferred until age ≥1 year. Children <4 months of age should not be vaccinated.)
- Pregnancy (Pregnant women who must travel to an area where the risk of yellow fever is high should be vaccinated when the risk of infection outweighs the theoretical risks of immunization.)
- Immunocompromised persons (including persons with HIV infection)
- Concurrent cholera and yellow fever vaccination impairs the immune response to each vaccine; these vaccines should be administered at a minimal interval of 3 weeks unless precluded by time constraints, when they should be given on the same day

Administration

- 0.5 mL subcutaneously (administered at least 10 days before the commencement of travel)
- International Health Regulations may require booster doses of 0.5 mL subcutaneously every 10 years

Vaccine Administration

Informed Consent and Documentation

Informed Consent

- Informed consent requirements are determined by state law
- Legal representative is defined as a parent or other individual who is qualified under state law to consent to the immunization of a minor
- The National Vaccine Injury Act of 1986 requires that the following information be provided:
  - Benefits of the vaccine
  - Risks associated with the vaccine
  - A statement of availability of the National Vaccine Injury Compensation Program

Instructions for Use of Vaccine Information Statements[1]

Required use of materials

- As required under the National Childhood Vaccine Injury Act (42 U.S.C. § 300aa-26), all health-care providers in the United States who administer any vaccine containing diphtheria, tetanus, pertussis, measles, mumps, rubella, or polio vaccine shall, before administration of *each dose* of the vaccine, provide a copy of the relevant vaccine information materials that have been produced by the Centers for Disease Control and Prevention (CDC):
  - To the parent or legal representative of any child to whom the provider intends to administer such vaccine, and
  - To any adult to whom the provider intends to administer such vaccine
- The materials shall be supplemented with visual presentations or oral explanations, in appropriate cases
- Additional recommended use of materials:
  - Health-care providers may also want to give parents

[1]The vaccine information statements are available on the Internet at www.vaccine.uthscsa.edu.

copies of all vaccine information materials before the first visit for immunization, such as at the first well baby visit
- Advised for other vaccines; providing information is required for hepatitis A, hepatitis B, and *Haemophilus influenzae* type b vaccines if purchased through federal contracts

Vaccine Record Keeping

- Health-care providers shall make a notation in each patient's permanent medical record (or in a permanent office log) at the time vaccine information materials are provided, indicating the following:
  - Date of administration
  - Name, address, and title of the individual who administers the vaccine
  - Vaccine manufacturer and lot number of the vaccine used
  - The edition (date of publication) of the materials distributed and the date the materials were provided
- Signed consent is not required by federal law but may be required by state law
- Adverse events, including those in the Vaccine Injury Table (page 124), must be reported (the law currently stipulates any penalties for failure to report)

Applicability of State Law

- Health-care providers should consult their legal counsel to determine additional state requirements pertaining to immunization; the federal requirement to provide the vaccine information materials supplements any applicable state law

General Guidelines for Vaccinations[1]

Vaccine Storage

- Most vaccines should be stored at 35°F–46°F (2°C–8°C); the notable exception is varicella vaccine (5°F [−15°C]; page 73)

Administration

- In general, inactivated vaccines are administered intramuscularly, and live-virus vaccines are administered subcutaneously; inactivated polio and pneumococcal vaccines may be given either intramuscularly or subcutaneously
- Vaccines administered by intramuscular injection should be given in the deltoid muscle or in the anterolateral aspect of the mid-thigh for children <24 months of age; some vaccines (e.g., HDCV) are contraindicated for intramuscular administration in the gluteal muscle
- Multiple vaccinations
  - If two or more vaccines or a vaccine and an immune globulin preparation are to be administered simultaneously, each is administered with a separate syringe, preferably at different anatomical sites into separate limbs. It is preferable to avoid administering two intramuscular injections in the same limb. If more than one intramuscular injection must be administered into a single limb, the thigh is usually the preferred site because of the greater muscle mass; the injections should be sufficiently separated (e.g., 1–2 inches apart) so that any local reactions are unlikely to overlap
  - Concurrent cholera and yellow fever vaccination impairs the immune response to each vaccine. These vaccines

[1]This information is based on the recommendations of the Advisory Committee on Immunization Practices (ACIP) and the Committee on Infectious Diseases (Red Book Committee) of the American Academy of Pediatrics (AAP). Sometimes these recommendations differ from those contained in the manufacturer's package inserts. For more detailed information, providers should consult the published recommendations of the ACIP and AAP and the manufacturer's package inserts.

should be administered at a minimal interval of 3 weeks unless precluded by time constraints, when they should be given on the same day
- MMR and varicella vaccines, if not given at the same time, should be given at least 30 days apart

Restarting Vaccination Series

- It is not necessary to restart the series of any childhood vaccine because of an extended interval between doses (the only exception is the oral typhoid vaccine)

Vaccination of Preterm Infants

- Infants born prematurely, regardless of birth weight, should be vaccinated at the same chronological age as full-term infants and children, except for low–birth weight premature infants of HBsAg-negative mothers (page 56)
- The full recommended dose of each vaccine should be used; divided or reduced doses are not recommended
- Administration of OPV, if used, should be deferred until hospital discharge to prevent the theoretical risk of poliovirus transmission in the hospital

Breast-feeding

- Breast-feeding does not adversely affect immunization and is not a contraindication for any vaccine
- Breast-fed infants should be vaccinated according to routine recommended schedules
- No vaccine (inactivated, killed-virus, or live-virus) affects the safety of breast-feeding for mothers or infants; breast-feeding mothers can continue breast-feeding without any interruption in the feeding schedule
  - Rubella vaccine virus may be transmitted in breast milk, but the virus does not usually infect the infant, and if infection does occur, it is well tolerated

Prevaccination Screening

- Prevaccination screening is likely to be cost effective for hepatitis A for persons >40 years of age as well as for younger persons in certain groups with a high prevalence of HAV infection

- Prevaccination screening may be recommended for hepatitis B depending on the specific level of risk and/or likelihood of previous exposure to HBV
- Prevaccination screening may be cost effective for varicella for adults since most adults are immune

General Contraindications[2]

- Anaphylactic reaction to a vaccine contraindicates further doses of that vaccine
- Anaphylactic reaction to a vaccine constituent contraindicates the use of vaccines containing that substance
- Moderate or severe illnesses with or without a fever

Not Contraindications

- Mild to moderate local reaction (soreness, redness, swelling) following a dose of an injectable antigen
- Mild acute illness with or without low-grade fever
- Current antimicrobial therapy
- Convalescent phase of illnesses
- Prematurity (same dosage and indications as for normal, full-term infants)
- Recent exposure to an infectious disease
- History of penicillin or other nonspecific allergies or family history of such allergies
- Breast-feeding

---

[2]Adapted from Centers for Disease Control and Prevention. General recommendations on immunization. Recommendations of the Advisory Committee on Immunization Practices (ACIP). *MMWR Morb Mortal Wkly Rep* 1994;43 (RR-1): 24–25.

Minimum Age for Initial Vaccination and Minimum Interval between Vaccine Doses[1]

Vaccine	Minimum Age for First Dose	Minimum Interval from Dose 1 to 2	Minimum Interval from Dose 2 to 3	Minimum Interval from Dose 3 to 4
Routine Childhood Vaccines				
Hepatitis B	Birth	1 month	2 months (≥4 months after dose 1)[6]	
DTP (or DT)[2]	6 weeks[3]	1 month	1 month	6 months
DTaP	6 weeks			
HbCV				
HbOC	6 weeks	1 month	1 month	2 months and at least 12 months of age[4]
PRP-T	6 weeks	1 month	1 month	2 months and at least 12 months of age[4]
PRP-OMP	6 weeks	1 month	2 months and at least 12 months of age[4]	No dose 4
Combined DTP/HbCV	6 weeks	1 month	1 month	6 months
OPV	6 weeks[3]	6 weeks	6 weeks	
IPV	6 weeks	1 month	6 months	
Rotavirus	6 weeks	3 weeks	3 weeks	
Measles or MMR	12 months[5]	1 month		
Varicella	12 months	1 month[7]		

Table continued on following page

Vaccine	Minimum Age for First Dose	Minimum Interval from Dose 1 to 2	Minimum Interval from Dose 2 to 3	Minimum Interval from Dose 3 to 4
Special Vaccines				
Hepatitis A				
Havrix	2 years	6 months		
Vaqta	2 years	6 months		
Influenza	6 months	1 month in children <9 years of age for the first series only; single dose annually thereafter		
Typhoid				
Vi capsular polysaccharide	2 years	Booster every 2 years		
Heat-phenol inactivated	6 months	4 weeks; booster every 3 years		
Oral live attenuated (Ty21a)	6 years	Booster (repeat series) every 5 years		
Japanese encephalitis	1 year	7 days	7 days	
Cholera	6 months	1 week		

One month is defined operationally as 28 days.

[1]See page 2 for recommended routine immunization schedule and page 6 for accelerated immunization schedule for children whose immunizations have been delayed.

[2]Children who have received all four primary vaccination doses before their fourth birthday should receive a fifth dose of DTP (or DT) or DTaP at 4–6 years of age before entering kindergarten or elementary school *and* at least 6 months after the fourth dose. The total number of doses of diphtheria and tetanus toxoids should not exceed six each before the seventh birthday.

[3]The American Academy of Pediatrics permits DTP and OPV to be administered as early as 4 weeks of age in areas with high endemicity and during outbreaks.

[4]The booster dose of Hib that is recommended following the primary vaccination series should be administered no earlier than 12 months of age *and* at least 2 months after the previous dose of Hib.

[5]Children in outbreak areas receiving initial measles vaccination <1 year of age should be revaccinated at 12–15 months of age, and an additional dose of vaccine should be administered at the time of school entry or according to local policy.

[6]The third dose of hepatitis B vaccine is recommended no earlier than 4 months of age.

[7]Only one dose of varicella vaccine is necessary for children 12 months to 13 years of age. Two doses are necessary for adolescents and adults ≥13 years of age.

General Guidelines for Spacing the Administration of Killed and Live Antigens

Antigen Combination	Recommended Minimum Interval Between Doses
≥2 killed antigens	No minimum; may be administered simultaneously or at any interval between doses[1]
Killed and live antigens	No minimum; may be administered simultaneously or at any interval between doses[2]
≥2 live antigens	4-week minimum interval if not administered simultaneously; however, oral polio vaccine (OPV) can be administered at any time before, with, or after measles-mumps-rubella, if indicated[3]

Adapted from Centers for Disease Control and Prevention. General recommendations on immunization. Recommendations of the Advisory Committee on Immunization Practices (ACIP). *MMWR Morb Mortal Wkly Rep* 1994;43 (RR-1):15.

[1]If possible, vaccines associated with local or systemic side effects (e.g., cholera, heat-phenol inactivated parenteral typhoid, and plague vaccines) should be administered on separate occasions to avoid accentuated reactions.

[2]The combination of yellow fever vaccine and cholera vaccine is the only exception. If time permits, these antigens should not be administered simultaneously, and at least 3 weeks should elapse between administration of yellow fever vaccine and cholera vaccine. If the vaccines must be administered simultaneously or within 3 weeks of each other, the antibody response may not be optimal.

[3]If oral live typhoid vaccine is indicated (e.g., for international travel undertaken on short notice), it can be administered before, simultaneously with, or after OPV.

Guidelines for Spacing the Administration of Immune Globulin Preparations[1] and Vaccines

Immunobiological Combination		Recommended Minimum Interval Between Doses
Simultaneous Administration		
Immune globulin and killed antigen		None; may be administered simultaneously or at any interval between doses[1]
Immune globulin and live virus		Should generally not be administered simultaneously[2]; if simultaneous administration of immune globulin with measles, mumps, and rubella (MMR), measles and rubella, monovalent measles vaccine, or varicella vaccine is unavoidable, administer at different sites and revaccinate or test for seroconversion after the recommended interval (page 112)
Nonsimultaneous Administration		
First	*Second*	
Immune globulin	Killed antigen	None
Killed antigen	Immune globulin	None
Immune globulin	Live virus	Dose related (page 112)[2,3]
Live virus	Immune globulin	2 weeks for MMR; 3 weeks for varicella vaccine

Adapted from Centers for Disease Control and Prevention. General recommendations on immunization. Recommendations of the Advisory Committee on Immunization Practices (ACIP). *MMWR Morb Mortal Wkly Rep* 1994;43 (RR-1):16.

[1]Blood products containing large amounts of immune globulin (e.g., immune globulin [IG] for intramuscular injection, specific immune globulins [e.g., TIG, HBIG, VZIG, RSV, IGIV], intravenous immune globulin [IVIG], whole blood, packed red blood cells, plasma, platelet products).

[2]Yellow fever, oral poliovirus, and oral typhoid (Ty21a) vaccines are exceptions to these recommendations. These vaccines may be administered at any time before, after, or simultaneously with an immune globulin–containing product without substantially decreasing the antibody response.

[3]The duration of interference of immune globulin preparations with the immune response to live virus vaccines is dose related (page 112).

Recommended Intervals between Administration of Immune Globulin Preparations or Blood Products and Vaccination with Preparations Containing Live Virus (Measles/MMR or Varicella)

Indication	Product, Dose, and Route	Equivalent IgG in mg/kg	Minimum Interval Before Vaccination (Months)[1]
Immunoprophylaxis			
Tetanus prophylaxis	TIG, 250 units intramuscularly	10	Measles: 3 Varicella: 5
Hepatitis A prophylaxis			
Contact prophylaxis	IG, 0.02 mL/kg intramuscularly	3.3	Measles: 3 Varicella: 5
International travel	IG, 0.06 mL/kg intramuscularly	10	Measles: 3 Varicella: 5
Hepatitis B prophylaxis	HBIG, 0.06 mL/kg intramuscularly	10	Measles: 3 Varicella: 5
Rabies prophylaxis	HRIG, 20 IU/kg intramuscularly	22	Measles: 4 Varicella: 5
Varicella prophylaxis	VZIG, 125 units/10 kg (maximum dose 625 units)	20–40	5
Measles prophylaxis			
Immunocompetent contact	IG, 0.25 mL/kg intramuscularly	40	5
Immunocompromised contact	IG, 0.50 mL/kg intramuscularly	80	6

RSV prophylaxis	RSV IGIV, 750 mg/kg intravenously	750	9
Immunoglobulin Replacement Therapy	IVIG, 300–400 mg/kg	300–400	8
Treatment of:			
Immune thrombocytopenic purpura (ITP)	IVIG, 400 mg/kg	400	8
	IVIG, 1000 mg/kg	1000	10
Kawasaki syndrome	IVIG, 2 g/kg	2000	11
Blood Transfusion			
Red blood cells, washed	10 mL/kg intravenously	Negligible	0
Red blood cells, adenine-saline added	10 mL/kg intravenously	10	3
Red blood cells, packed	10 mL/kg intravenously	60	6
Whole blood	10 mL/kg intravenously	80–100	6
Platelets	10 mL/kg intravenously	160	7
Plasma	10 mL/kg intravenously	160	7

Adapted from Centers for Disease Control and Prevention. General recommendations on immunization. Recommendations of the Advisory Committee on Immunization Practices (ACIP). *MMWR Morb Mortal Wkly Rep* 1994;43 (RR-1):17.

[1]If an immune globulin preparation or blood product is given in the interval before measles or varicella vaccination is recommended, the recipient should be revaccinated at or after the appropriate interval unless serological testing indicates that measles- or varicella-specific antibodies are induced.

Algorithm for Testing and Desensitization for Vaccinating Patients with Hypersensitivity to Eggs and Egg Products[1]

History consistent with egg allergy[2]:

- Urticaria
- Angioedema
- Nausea or vomiting
- Diarrhea
- Abdominal pain
- Stridor
- Wheezing
- Hypotension with tachycardia

} Within 2 hours of egg ingestion

↓

Prick test with vaccine diluted 1:10 in normal saline

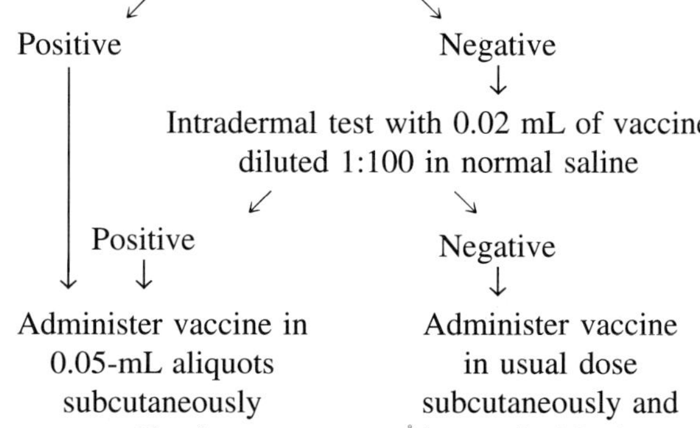

Adapted from protocols from Herman JJ, Radin R, Schneiderman R: Allergic reactions to measles (rubeola) vaccine in patients hypersensitive to egg protein. *J Pediatr* 1983;102:196–199; Greenberg MA, Birx DL: Safe administration of mumps-measles-rubella vaccine in egg-allergic children. *J Pediatr* 1988:113:504–506.

[1]Vaccines prepared using embryonated chicken eggs include influenza and yellow fever vaccines. Vaccines prepared using chicken egg embryo cell cultures include measles and mumps (and MMR). Most anaphylactic reactions to measles and mumps vaccines are to gelatin or other components. No specific protocols for skin testing to gelatin have been established.

[2]Generally, persons who are able to eat eggs or egg products without adverse effects may receive these vaccines. Persons with histories of anaphylactic hypersensitivity (e.g., urticaria, swelling of the mouth and throat, difficulty breathing, hypotension, or shock) to eggs or egg proteins should not receive these vaccines.

Licensed Vaccines and Toxoids Available in the United States

Vaccine	Trade Name	Manufacturer	Type	Route of Administration
Vaccines against Bacteria				
Bacillus anthracis (anthrax)[1]	Anthrax Vaccine, Absorbed	Michigan BPI	Inactivated bacteria	Subcutaneous
Bacille Calmette-Guérin (BCG)	Tice BCG	Organon Teknika	Live bacteria ($1–8 \times 10^8$ CFU/mL)	Percutaneous/intradermal[2]
Bordetella pertussis (pertussis)	Pertussis Vaccine, Adsorbed	Michigan BPI	Inactivated whole *B. pertussis* (4 units)	
Clostridium tetani (tetanus)	TE Anatoxal Berna	Berna	Inactivated toxin (toxoid) (10 Lf/0.5 mL)	Intramuscular
	Tetanus Toxoid, Adsorbed	Connaught	Inactivated toxin (toxoid) (5 Lf/0.5 mL)	Intramuscular
	Tetanus Toxoid, Adsorbed	Wyeth-Lederle	Inactivated toxin (toxoid) (5 Lf/0.5 mL)	Intramuscular
	Tetanus Toxoid, Adsorbed	Massachusetts PHBL	Inactivated toxin (toxoid) (5 Lf/0.5 mL)	Intramuscular
	Tetanus Toxoid, Adsorbed	Michigan BPI	Inactivated toxin (toxoid) (5–10 Lf/0.5 mL)	Intramuscular
	Tetanus Toxoid, Adsorbed	Wyeth-Ayerst	Inactivated toxin (toxoid) (5 Lf/0.5 mL)	Intramuscular
	Tetanus Toxoid, Fluid	Connaught	Inactivated toxin (toxoid)	Intramuscular
	Tetanus Toxoid, Fluid	Wyeth-Lederle		
	Tetanus Toxoid, Fluid	Sclavo SpA		
	Tetanus Toxoid, Fluid	Wyeth-Ayerst		

Table continued on following page

Vaccine	Trade Name	Manufacturer	Type	Route of Administration
Haemophilus influenzae type b (page 55)	PedvaxHIB	Merck	Bacterial capsular polysaccharide (15 μg/0.5 mL) conjugated to OMP (an outer membrane protein complex of group B *Neisseria meningitidis*)	Intramuscular
	HibTITER	Wyeth-Lederle	Bacterial capsular oligosaccharide (10 μg/0.5 mL) conjugated to CRM_{197} (a non-toxic naturally occurring mutant of diphtheria toxin)	
	ActHIB (same as OmniHIB)	Pasteur Mérieux Connaught	Bacterial capsular polysaccharide (10 μg/0.5 mL) conjugated to tetanus toxoid	
	OmniHIB (same as ActHIB)	SmithKline Beecham	Bacterial capsular polysaccharide (10 μg/0.5 mL) conjugated to tetanus toxoid	
	ProHIBit	Connaught	Bacterial capsular polysaccharide (25 μg/0.5 mL) conjugated to diphtheria toxoid	
Salmonella typhi (typhoid)	Typhim Vi	Connaught	Polysaccharide antigen (25 μg/0.5 mL)	Intramuscular
	Typhoid Vaccine, USP	Wyeth-Ayerst	Inactivated (heat-phenol) bacteria (strain Ty2) (≤1 billion organisms/mL)	Subcutaneous[4]
	Vivotif Berna	Swiss Serum and Vaccine Institute	Live-attenuated *S. typhi* strain Ty21a ($2–6 \times 10^6$ CFU of viable *S. typhi* organisms per capsule, plus $5–50 \times 10^9$ nonviable bacterial cells)	Oral
	Typhoid Vaccine, USP[1]	Wyeth-Ayerst	Inactivated (acetone inactivated, dried) bacteria (strain Ty2) (≤1 billion organisms/mL)	Subcutaneous

Streptococcus pneumoniae (pneumococcus)	Pneumovax 23 Pnu-Immune 23	Merck Wyeth-Lederle	Capsular polysaccharides of 23 pneumococcal serotypes (25 μg of each serotype/0.5 mL)	Intramuscular or subcutaneous
Neisseria meningitidis (meningococcus)	Menomune-A/C/Y/W-135	Pasteur Mérieux Connaught	Capsular polysaccharides of serotypes A, C, Y, and W-135 (50 μg of each serotype/0.5 mL)	Subcutaneous
Vibrio cholerae (cholera)	Generic	Wyeth-Ayerst	Inactivated bacteria (4 billion bacteria of each Ogawa [NIH 41] and Inaba [NIH 35A3] serotype/mL)	Subcutaneous or intradermal[5]
Yersinia pestis (plague)	Plague Vaccine	Cutter	Inactivated bacteria ($1.8–2.2 \times 10^8$ bacteria/mL)	Intramuscular
Vaccines against Viruses				
Adenovirus[1]				
Adenovirus type 4	Generic	Wyeth-Ayerst	Live virus (≥32,000 $TCID_{50}$ [$10^{4.5}$ TCID]/tablet)	Oral
Adenovirus type 7	Generic	Wyeth-Ayerst	Live virus (≥32,000 $TCID_{50}$ [$10^{4.5}$ TCID]/tablet)	Oral
Hepatitis A	Havrix	SmithKline Beecham	Inactivated virus	Intramuscular
	Vaqta	Merck	Inactivated virus	Intramuscular
Hepatitis B	Engerix-B	SmithKline Beecham	Inactive viral antigen	Intramuscular
	Recombivax HB	Merck	Inactive viral antigen	Intramuscular

Table continued on following page

Vaccine	Trade Name	Manufacturer	Type	Route of Administration
Influenza	Fluzone	Pasteur Mérieux Connaught	Inactivated whole virus (for adults only) or subvirion (split) virus components (adults and children) (15 μg of each strain/0.5 mL, reformulated annually)	Intramuscular
	FluShield	Wyeth-Ayerst	Split virus components (15 μg of each strain/0.5 mL, reformulated annually)	Intramuscular
	Fluvirin	Evans/Medeva[3]	Purified surface antigen (15 μg of each strain/0.5 mL, reformulated annually)	Intramuscular
Japanese encephalitis	JE-Vax	Biken/Pasteur Mérieux Connaught[3]	Inactivated virus (2–3 μg total nitrogen/mL)	Subcutaneous
Measles	Attenuvax	Merck	Live-attenuated virus (≥1,000 $TCID_{50}$/dose of Moraten strain)	Subcutaneous
Mumps	Mumpsvax	Merck	Live-attenuated virus (≥20,000 $TCID_{50}$/dose of Jeryl-Lynn strain)	Subcutaneous
Poliovirus (polio)	Orimune	Wyeth-Lederle	Live-attenuated viruses of all 3 serotypes (type 1—$10^{5.4\text{-}6.4}$, type 2—$10^{4.5\text{-}5.5}$, type 3—$10^{5.2\text{-}6.2}$; comparable to 800,000, 100,000, and 500,000 viral particles, respectively, per 0.5 mL)	Oral
	IPOL, Poliovax	Pasteur Mérieux Connaught	Inactivated viruses of all 3 serotypes grown in monkey kidney cells (IPOL) or human fibroblast (MRC-5) cells (Poliovax) (40, 8, and 32 D-antigen units of types 1, 2, and 3, respectively, per 0.5 mL)	Subcutaneous or intramuscular

Rabies	Imovax-Rabies	Pasteur Mérieux Connaught	Inactivated virus (Pitman Moore strain [PM-1503-3M]) prepared in human cells	Intramuscular
	Imovax-Rabies I.D.	Pasteur Mérieux Connaught	Inactivated virus (Pitman Moore strain [PM-1503-3M]) prepared in human cells	Intradermal[6]
	RabAvert	Chiron Behring GmbH	Inactivated virus (Flury strain) prepared in chicken embryo fibroblasts	Intramuscular
	Rabies Vaccine, Adsorbed	Michigan BPI/ SmithKline Beecham[3]	Inactivated virus (Kissling strain) prepared in fetal Rhesus lung cells	Intramuscular
Rotavirus	RotaShield	Wyeth-Lederle	Live-attenuated quadrivalent (1×10^5 PFU of each: Rhesus rotavirus G3 and human-Rhesus G1 [DxRRV], G2 [DS1xRRV], and G4 [ST3xRRV])	Oral
Rubella	Meruvax II	Merck	Live-attenuated virus (≥1000 $TCID_{50}$/dose of RA27/3 strain)	Subcutaneous
Smallpox	Dryvax	Wyeth-Ayerst (available only from the CDC)	Live-attenuated virus (2.5×10^5 PFU/dose)	Scarification
Varicella-zoster virus (chickenpox)	Varivax	Merck	Live-attenuated virus (≥3300 PFU/dose at time of manufacture [1350 PFU/dose after reconstitution at the expiration date, of Oka strain])	Subcutaneous (over the deltoid)
Yellow fever	YF-Vax	Pasteur Mérieux Connaught	Live-attenuated virus (≥5.04 $\log_{10}$ PFU/0.5 mL ≥2000 mouse LD_{50} units)	Subcutaneous

Table continued on following page

Vaccine	Trade Name	Manufacturer	Type	Route of Administration
Combination Vaccines				
Diphtheria, tetanus, and pertussis (DTP)	Generic	Pasteur Mérieux Connaught	Diphtheria and tetanus toxoids and inactivated whole-cell *B. pertussis* (page 50)	Intramuscular
	Generic	Massachusetts PHBL		
	Generic	Michigan BPI/ SmithKline Beecham[3]		
	Tri-Immunol	Wyeth-Lederle		
Diphtheria, tetanus, and acellular pertussis (DTaP)	Acel-Imune	Wyeth-Lederle	Diphtheria and tetanus toxoids and inactivated *B. pertussis* components (page 50)	Intramuscular
	Certiva	North American Vaccine/Ross[3]		
	Infanrix	SmithKline Beecham		
	Tripedia	Pasteur Mérieux Connaught		
	(unnamed)[7]	Chiron-Biocine		

Diphtheria and tetanus (TD,[8] Td[8])	Generic	Connaught Wyeth-Lederle Massachusetts PHBL Michigan BPI Sclavo SpA Wyeth-Ayerst	Inactivated toxins (toxoids) (page 50)	Intramuscular
Diphtheria, tetanus, and pertussis with *Haemophilus influenzae* type b	Tetramune	Wyeth-Lederle	Diphtheria and tetanus toxoids, inactivated whole-cell pertussis, and *H. influenzae* type b polysaccharide conjugated to protein (HbOC [HibTITER])	Intramuscular
	TriHIBit	Pasteur Mérieux Connaught (ActHIB reconstituted with Tripedia [DTaP])	*Haemophilus influenzae* type b conjugate vaccine (ActHIB) combined by reconstitution with DTaP (Tripedia)	Intramuscular
Haemophilus influenzae type b and hepatitis B	Comvax	Merck	*Haemophilus influenzae* type b (7.5 μg PRP-OMP [PedvaxHIB]) and 5 μg hepatitis B (Recombivax HB)	Intramuscular

Table continued on following page

Vaccine	Trade Name	Manufacturer	Type	Route of Administration
Measles, mumps, and rubella	M-M-R II	Merck	Live-attenuated virus Measles: 1000 $TCID_{50}$/dose of Moraten strain Mumps: 20,000 $TCID_{50}$/dose of Jeryl-Lynn strain Rubella: 1000 $TCID_{50}$/dose of RA27/3 strain	Subcutaneous
Measles and rubella	M-R-Vax II	Merck	Live-attenuated virus Measles: 1000 $TCID_{50}$/dose of Moraten strain Rubella: 1000 $TCID_{50}$/dose of RA27/3 strain	Subcutaneous
Mumps and rubella	Biavax II	Merck	Live-attenuated virus Mumps: 20,000 $TCID_{50}$/dose of Jeryl-Lynn strain Rubella: 1000 $TCID_{50}$/dose of RA27/3 strain	Subcutaneous

[1]Available only to the U.S. Armed Forces.

[2]Tice BCG and another BCG preparation, TheraCys (Connaught), are licensed for intravesical instillation for prophylaxis against recurrent papillary carcinoma of the urinary bladder. TheraCys is not intended to be used as an immunizing agent for prevention of tuberculosis.

[3]Manufacturer/distributor.

[4]Booster doses may be administered intradermally (page 91).

[5]The intradermal dose is lower than the subcutaneous dose.

[6]The intradermal dose of human diploid cell (HDCV) rabies vaccine is lower than the intramuscular dose and is used only for preexposure vaccination. Rabies vaccine, adsorbed (RVA) should not be used intradermally.

[7]FDA approval is pending as of September 1, 1998.

[8]*TD*, Tetanus and diphtheria toxoids for use among children <7 years of age; *Td*, tetanus and diphtheria toxoids for use among persons ≥7 years of age. Td contains the same amount of tetanus toxoid as DTP or DT but contains a smaller dose of diphtheria toxoid.

Reportable Adverse Events Following Vaccination

Vaccines Included

- Mandatory reporting
  - DTP, DT, Td, tetanus, pertussis, OPV, eIPV, measles, mumps, rubella
  - Events listed in the Vaccine Injury Table (Reportable Events Table)
- Voluntary reporting
  - All other vaccines
  - Serious adverse events felt to be related to vaccination but not listed in the Vaccine Injury Table

How to Report

- Health-care providers, vaccine recipients, or parents or guardians of vaccine recipients
- Complete the VAERS form and submit as indicated (the VAERS form is available on the Internet at www.vaccine.uthscsa.edu)

National Vaccine Injury Compensation Program Vaccine Injury Table[1]

Vaccine	Illness, Disability, Injury or Condition Covered	Time Lapse until Appearance of First Symptom or Manifestation of Onset or of Significant Aggravation after Vaccine Administration
Vaccines containing tetanus toxoid (e.g., DTaP, DTP, DT, Td, or TT)	Anaphylaxis or anaphylactic shock	4 hours
	Brachial neuritis	2–28 days
	Any acute complication or sequela (including death) of an illness, disability, injury, or condition referred to above which illness, disability, injury, or condition arose within the time period prescribed	Not applicable
Vaccines containing whole-cell pertussis bacteria, extracted or partial-cell pertussis bacteria, or specific pertussis antigen(s) (e.g., DTaP, DTP, P, DTP-Hib)	Anaphylaxis or anaphylactic shock	4 hours
	Encephalopathy (or encephalitis)	72 hours
	Any acute complication or sequela (including death) of an illness, disability, injury, or condition referred to above which illness, disability, injury, or condition arose within the time period prescribed	Not applicable

[1]Effective date: March 24, 1997.

Table continued on following page

Vaccine	Illness, Disability, Injury or Condition Covered	Time Lapse until Appearance of First Symptom or Manifestation of Onset or of Significant Aggravation after Vaccine Administration
Measles, mumps, and rubella vaccine or any of its components (e.g., MMR, MR, M, R)	Anaphylaxis or anaphylactic shock	4 hours
	Encephalopathy (or encephalitis)	5–15 days (not less than 5 days and not more than 15 days) for measles, mumps, rubella, or any vaccine containing any of the foregoing as a component
	Any acute complication or sequela (including death) of an illness, disability, injury, or condition referred to above which illness, disability, injury, or condition arose within the time period prescribed	Not applicable
Vaccines containing rubella virus (e.g., MMR, MR, R)	Chronic arthritis	7–42 days
	Any acute complication or sequela (including death) of an illness, disability, injury, or condition referred to above which illness, disability, injury, or condition arose within the time period prescribed	Not applicable

Vaccine	Illness, Disability, Injury or Condition Covered	Time Lapse until Appearance of First Symptom or Manifestation of Onset or of Significant Aggravation after Vaccine Administration
Vaccines containing measles virus (e.g., MMR, MR, M)	Thrombocytopenic purpura	7–30 days
	Vaccine-strain measles viral infection in an immunodeficient recipient	6 months
	Any acute complication or sequela (including death) of an illness, disability, injury, or condition referred to above which illness, disability, injury, or condition arose within the time period prescribed	Not applicable
Vaccines containing polio live virus (OPV)	Paralytic polio	
	In a nonimmunodeficient recipient	30 days
	In an immunodeficient recipient	6 months
	In a vaccine-associated community case	Not applicable

Table continued on following page

Vaccine	Illness, Disability, Injury or Condition Covered	Time Lapse until Appearance of First Symptom or Manifestation of Onset or of Significant Aggravation after Vaccine Administration
Vaccines containing polio live virus *Continued*	Vaccine-strain polio viral infection	
	In a nonimmunodeficient recipient	30 days
	In an immunodeficient recipient	6 months
	In a vaccine-associated community case	Not applicable
	Any acute complication or sequela (including death) of an illness, disability, injury, or condition referred to above which illness, disability, injury, or condition arose within the time period prescribed	Not applicable

Vaccine	Illness, Disability, Injury or Condition Covered	Time Lapse until Appearance of First Symptom or Manifestation of Onset or of Significant Aggravation after Vaccine Administration
Vaccines containing polio inactivated virus (e.g., IPV)	Anaphylaxis or anaphylactic shock	4 hours
	Any acute complication or sequela (including death) of an illness, disability, injury, or condition referred to above which illness, disability, injury, or condition arose within the time period prescribed	Not applicable
Hepatitis B vaccines	Anaphylaxis or anaphylactic shock	4 hours
	Any acute complication or sequela (including death) of an illness, disability, injury, or condition referred to above which illness, disability, injury, or condition arose within the time period prescribed	Not applicable

Table continued on following page

Vaccine	Illness, Disability, Injury or Condition Covered	Time Lapse until Appearance of First Symptom or Manifestation of Onset or of Significant Aggravation after Vaccine Administration
Haemophilus influenzae type b polysaccharide vaccines (unconjugated, PRP vaccines)	Early-onset Hib disease	7 days
	Any acute complication or sequela (including death) of an illness, disability, injury, or condition referred to above when the illness, disability, injury, or condition arose within the time period prescribed	Not applicable
Haemophilus influenzae type b polysaccharide conjugate vaccines	No condition specified	Not applicable
Varicella vaccine	No condition specified	Not applicable
Any new vaccine recommended by the Centers for Disease Control and Prevention for routine administration to children, after publication by the secretary of a notice of coverage	No condition specified	Not applicable

QUALIFICATIONS AND AIDS TO INTERPRETATION

I Anaphylaxis and Anaphylactic Shock

Anaphylaxis and anaphylactic shock mean an acute, severe, and potentially lethal systemic allergic reaction. Most cases resolve without sequelae. Signs and symptoms begin minutes to a few hours after exposure. Death, if it occurs, usually results from airway obstruction caused by laryngeal edema or bronchospasm and may be associated with cardiovascular collapse. Other significant clinical signs and symptoms may include the following: cyanosis, hypotension, bradycardia, tachycardia, dysrhythmia, edema of the pharynx and/or trachea and/or larynx with stridor and dyspnea. Autopsy findings may include acute emphysema, which results from lower respiratory tract obstruction; edema of the hypopharynx, epiglottis, larynx, or trachea; and minimal findings of eosinophilia in the liver, spleen, and lungs. When death occurs within minutes of exposure and without signs of respiratory distress, there may not be significant pathological findings.

II Encephalopathy

For purposes of the Vaccine Injury Table, a vaccine recipient shall be considered to have suffered an encephalopathy only if such recipient manifests, within the applicable period, an injury meeting the description below of an acute encephalopathy, and then a chronic encephalopathy persists in such person for more than 6 months beyond the date of vaccination.

A. An acute encephalopathy is one that is sufficiently severe to require hospitalization (whether or not hospitalization occurred).
   1. For children younger than 18 months of age who present without an associated seizure event, an acute encephalopathy is indicated by a "significantly decreased level of consciousness" (see paragraph 4 below) lasting for at least 24 hours. Those children younger than 18 months of age who present following a seizure shall be viewed as having an acute encephalopathy if their significantly decreased level of consciousness persists beyond 24

hours and cannot be attributed to a postictal state (seizure) or medication.

2. For adults and children 18 months of age or older, an acute encephalopathy is one that persists for at least 24 hours and is characterized by at least two of the following:
   a. A significant change in mental status that is not medication related; specifically a confusional state, or a delirium, or a psychosis;
   b. A significantly decreased level of consciousness, which is independent of a seizure and cannot be attributed to the effects of medication; and
   c. A seizure associated with loss of consciousness.
3. Increased intracranial pressure may be a clinical feature of acute encephalopathy in any age group.
4. A significantly decreased level of consciousness is indicated by the presence of at least one of the following clinical signs for at least 24 hours or greater (see paragraphs II, A, 1 and II, A, 2 of this section for applicable time frames):
   a. Decreased or absent response to environment (responds, if at all, only to loud voice or painful stimuli);
   b. Decreased or absent eye contact (does not fix gaze on family members or other individuals); or
   c. Inconsistent or absent responses to external stimuli (does not recognize familiar people or things).
5. The following clinical features alone, or in combination, do not demonstrate an acute encephalopathy or a significant change in either mental status or level of consciousness as described above: sleepiness, irritability (fussiness), high-pitched and unusual screaming, persistent inconsolable crying, and bulging fontanelle. Seizures in themselves are not sufficient to constitute a diagnosis of encephalopathy. In the absence of other evidence of an acute encephalopathy, seizures shall not be viewed as the first symptom or manifestation of the onset of an acute encephalopathy.

B. Chronic encephalopathy occurs when a change in mental or neurological status, first manifested during the applicable time period, persists for a period of at least 6 months from the date of vaccination. Individuals who return to a normal neurological state after the acute encephalopathy shall not be presumed to have suffered residual neurological damage from that event; any subsequent chronic encephalopathy shall not be presumed to be a sequela of the acute encephalopathy. If a preponderance of the evidence indicates that a child's chronic encephalopathy is secondary to genetic, prenatal, or perinatal factors, that chronic encephalopathy shall not be considered to be a condition set forth in the Vaccine Injury Table.

C. An encephalopathy shall not be considered to be a condition set forth in the Vaccine Injury Table if in a proceeding on a petition, it is shown by a preponderance of the evidence that the encephalopathy was caused by an infection, a toxin, a metabolic disturbance, a structural lesion, a genetic disorder, or trauma (without regard to whether the cause of the infection, toxin, trauma, metabolic disturbance, structural lesion, or genetic disorder is known). If at the time a decision is made on a petition filed under section 2111(b) of the act for a vaccine-related injury or death, it is not possible to determine the cause by a preponderance of the evidence of an encephalopathy, the encephalopathy shall be considered to be a condition set forth in the Vaccine Injury Table.

D. In determining whether an encephalopathy is a condition set forth in the Vaccine Injury Table, the court shall consider the entire medical record.

III Residual Seizure Disorder

A petitioner may be considered to have suffered a residual seizure disorder for purposes of the Vaccine Injury Table if the first seizure or convulsion occurred 5–15 days (not less than 5 days and not more than 15 days) after administration of the vaccine and 2 or more additional distinct seizure or convulsion episodes occurred within 1 year after the administration of the vaccine that were unaccompanied by fever (defined as a rectal temperature equal to or greater than 101.0°F or an oral temperature equal to or greater than 100.0°F). A distinct seizure or convulsion episode is ordinarily defined as including all seizure or convulsive activity occurring within a 24-hour period, unless competent and qualified expert neurological testimony is presented to the contrary in a particular case.

For purposes of the Vaccine Injury Table, a petitioner shall not be considered to have suffered a residual seizure disorder if the petitioner suffered a seizure or convulsion unaccompanied by fever (as defined above) before the fifth day after the administration of the vaccine involved.

IV Seizure and Convulsion

For purposes of paragraphs II and III of this section, the terms "seizure" and "convulsion" include myoclonic, generalized tonic-clonic (grand mal), and simple and complex partial seizures. Absence (petit mal) seizures shall not be considered to be a condition set forth in the Vaccine Injury Table. Jerking movements or staring episodes alone are not necessarily an indication of seizure activity.

V Sequela

The term "sequela" means a condition or event that was actually caused by a condition listed in the Vaccine Injury Table.

VI Chronic Arthritis

For purposes of the Vaccine Injury Table, chronic arthritis may be found in a person with no history in the 3 years before vaccination of arthropathy (joint disease) on the basis of the following:

A. Medical documentation, recorded within 30 days after the onset, of objective signs of acute arthritis (joint swelling) that occurred between 7 and 42 days after a rubella vaccination;
B. Medical documentation (recorded within 3 years after the onset of acute arthritis) of the persistence of objective signs of intermittent or continuous arthritis for more than 6 months following vaccination; and
C. Medical documentation of an antibody response to the rubella virus.

For purposes of the Vaccine Injury Table, the following shall not be considered chronic arthritis: musculoskeletal disorders such as diffuse connective tissue diseases (including but not limited to rheumatoid arthritis, juvenile rheumatoid arthritis, systemic lupus erythematosus, systemic sclerosis, mixed connective tissue disease, polymyositis/dermatomyositis, fibromyalgia, necrotizing vasculitis and vasculopathies, and Sjögren syndrome), degenerative joint disease, infectious agents other than rubella (whether by direct invasion or as an immune reaction), metabolic and endocrine diseases, trauma, neoplasms, neuropathic disorders, bone and cartilage disorders and arthritis associated with ankylosing spondylitis, psoriasis, inflammatory bowel disease, Reiter syndrome, or blood disorders.

Arthralgia (joint pain) or stiffness without joint swelling shall not be viewed as chronic arthritis for purposes of the Vaccine Injury Table.

VII Brachial Neuritis

Brachial neuritis is defined as dysfunction limited to the upper extremity nerve plexus (i.e., its trunks, divisions, or cords) without involvement of other peripheral (e.g., nerve roots or a single peripheral nerve) or central (e.g., spinal cord) nervous system structures. A deep, steady, often severe aching pain in the shoulder and upper arm usually heralds onset of the condition. The pain is followed in days or weeks by weakness and atrophy in upper extremity muscle groups. Sensory loss may accompany the motor deficits but is generally a less notable clinical feature. The neuritis, or plexopathy, may be present on the same side or the opposite side of the injection; it is sometimes bilateral, affecting both upper extremities. Weakness is required before the diagnosis can be made. Motor, sensory, and reflex findings on physical examination and the results of nerve conduction and electromyographic studies must be consistent in confirming that dysfunction is attributable to the brachial plexus. The condition should thereby be distinguishable from conditions that may give rise to dysfunction of nerve roots (i.e., radiculopathies) and peripheral nerves (i.e., including multiple mononeuropathies), as well as other peripheral and central nervous system structures (e.g., cranial neuropathies and myelopathies).

VIII Thrombocytopenic Purpura

Thrombocytopenic purpura is defined by a serum platelet count less than 50,000/mm^3. Thrombocytopenic purpura does not include cases of thrombocytopenia associated with other causes, such as hypersplenism, autoimmune disorders (including alloantibodies from previous transfusions), myelodysplasias, lymphoproliferative disorders, congenital thrombocytopenia, or hemolytic uremic syndrome. It does not include cases of immune (formerly called idiopathic) thrombocytopenic purpura (ITP) that are mediated, for example, by viral or fungal infections, toxins, or drugs. Thrombocytopenic purpura does not include cases of thrombocytopenia associated with disseminated intravascular coagulation, as observed with bacterial and viral infections. Viral infections include, for example, those infections secondary to Epstein-Barr virus, cytomegalovirus, hepatitis A and B, rhinovirus, human immunodeficiency virus (HIV), adenovirus, and dengue virus. An antecedent viral infection may be demonstrated by clinical signs and symptoms and need not be confirmed by culture or serological testing. Bone marrow examination, if performed, must reveal a normal or an increased number of megakaryocytes in an otherwise normal marrow.

IX Vaccine-Strain Measles Viral Infection

Vaccine-strain measles viral infection is defined as a disease caused by the vaccine strain that should be determined by vaccine-specific monoclonal antibody or polymerase chain reaction tests.

X Vaccine-Strain Polio Viral Infection

Vaccine-strain polio viral infection is defined as a disease caused by poliovirus that is isolated from the affected tissue and should be determined to be the vaccine strain by oligonucleotide or polymerase chain reaction. Isolation of poliovirus from the stool is not sufficient to establish a tissue-specific infection or disease caused by vaccine-strain poliovirus.

XI Early-Onset Hib Disease

Early-onset Hib disease is defined as an invasive bacterial illness associated with the presence of Hib organism on culture of normally sterile body fluids or tissue, or clinical findings consistent with the diagnosis of epiglottitis. Hib pneumonia qualifies as invasive Hib disease when radiographic findings consistent with the diagnosis of pneumonitis are accompanied by a blood culture positive for the Hib organism. Otitis media, in the absence of the above findings, does not qualify as invasive bacterial disease. A child is considered to have acquired this injury only if the vaccine was the first Hib immunization received by the child.

Summarized Conclusions of Evidence Regarding the Possible Association between Specific Adverse Effects and Receipt of Childhood Vaccines by Determination of Causality

DTP Vaccine	DT/Td/ Tetanus Toxoid	Measles Vaccine[1]	Mumps Vaccine[1]	RA27/3 MMR[1,2]	OPV/IPV[3]	Hepatitis B Vaccine	*Haemophilus influenzae* type b Vaccine
No Evidence Available to Establish a Causal Relationship							
Autism	None	None	Neuropathy Residual seizure disorder	None	Transverse myelitis *(IPV)* Thrombocytopenia *(IPV)* Anaphylaxis *(IPV)*	None	None
Inadequate Evidence to Accept or Reject a Causal Relationship							
Aseptic meningitis Chronic neurological damage Erythema multiforme or other rash Guillain-Barré syndrome	Residual seizure disorder other than infantile spasms Demyelinating diseases of the central nervous system	Encephalopathy Subacute sclerosing panencephalitis Residual seizure disorder Optic neuritis	Encephalopathy Aseptic meningitis Insulin-dependent diabetes mellitus Sterility	Radiculoneuritis and other neuropathies Thrombocytopenic purpura Sensorineural deafness	Transverse myelitis *(OPV)* Guillain-Barré syndrome *(IPV)* Death from SIDS[5]	Guillain-Barré syndrome Demyelinating diseases of the central nervous system Arthritis Death from SIDS[5]	Guillain-Barré syndrome Transverse myelitis Thrombocytopenia Anaphylaxis Death from SIDS

Hemolytic anemia Juvenile diabetes Learning disabilities and attention-deficit disorder Peripheral mononeuropathy Thrombocytopenia	Mononeuropathy Arthritis Erythema multiforme	Transverse myelitis Guillain-Barré syndrome Thrombocytopenia Insulin-dependent diabetes mellitus	Thrombocytopenia Anaphylaxis[4]				
Evidence Favored Rejection of a Causal Relationship							
Infantile spasms Hypsarrhythmia Reye syndrome SIDS	Encephalopathy Infantile spasms (DT only)[6] Death from SIDS (DT only)[6,7]	None	None	None	None	None	Early onset *H. influenzae* type b disease (conjugate vaccines)

Table continued on following page

DTP Vaccine	DT/Td/ Tetanus Toxoid	Measles Vaccine[1]	Mumps Vaccine[1]	RA27/3 MMR[1,2]	OPV/IPV[3]	Hepatitis B Vaccine	*Haemophilus influenzae* type b Vaccine
Evidence Favored Acceptance of a Causal Relationship							
Acute encephalopathy[8] Shock and unusual shocklike state	Guillain-Barré syndrome[9,10] Brachial neuritis[9]	Anaphylaxis[4]	None	Chronic arthritis	Guillain-Barré syndrome *(OPV)*	None	Early-onset *H. influenzae* type b disease in children ≥18 months of age whose first Hib vaccination was with unconjugated PRP vaccine

Evidence Established a Causal Relationship							
Anaphylaxis Protracted, inconsolable crying	Anaphylaxis[9]	Death from measles-vaccine-strain viral infection[5,11]	None	Acute arthritis Thrombocytopenia Anaphylaxis[4]	Poliomyelitis in contact or recipient *(OPV)* Death from polio-vaccine-strain viral infection[5,11]	Anaphylaxis	None

This table is an adaptation of tables published in 1991 and 1994 by the Institute of Medicine (IOM), an independent research organization chartered by the National Academy of Sciences. The National Childhood Vaccine Injury Act of 1986 mandated that IOM review scientific and other evidence (e.g., epidemiological studies, case series, individual case reports, testimonials) regarding the possible adverse consequences of vaccines administered to children. IOM constituted an expert committee to review and summarize all available information; this committee created five categories of causality to describe the relationships between the vaccines and specific adverse events.

SIDS, Sudden infant death syndrome.

[1]If the data derived from studies of a monovalent preparation, then the causal relationship also extended to multivalent preparations (e.g., MMR). In the absence of data concerning the monovalent preparation, the causal relationship determined for the multivalent preparations did not extend to the monovalent components.

[2]Trivalent MMR vaccine containing the RA27/3 rubella strain.

[3]For some adverse events, the IOM committee was charged with assessing the causal relationship between the adverse event and only oral poliovirus vaccine (OPV) (i.e., for poliomyelitis) or only inactivated poliovirus vaccine (IPV) (i.e., for anaphylaxis and thrombocytopenia). If the conclusions for the two vaccines differed for the other adverse events, the vaccine to which the adverse event applied is specified parenthetically in italics.

Table continued on following page

[4]The evidence used to establish a causal relationship for anaphylaxis applies to MMR vaccine. The evidence regarding monovalent measles vaccine favored acceptance of a causal relationship, but this evidence was less convincing than that for MMR vaccine because of either incomplete documentation of symptoms or the possible attenuation of symptoms by medical intervention.

[5]This table lists weight-of-evidence determinations only for deaths that were classified as sudden infant death syndrome (SIDS) and deaths that were a consequence of vaccine-strain viral infection. However, if the evidence favored the acceptance of (or established) a causal relationship between a vaccine and a possibly fatal adverse event, then the evidence also favored the acceptance of (or established) a causal relationship between the vaccine and death from the adverse event. Direct evidence regarding death in association with a vaccine-associated adverse event was limited to (1) Td and Guillain-Barré syndrome, (2) tetanus toxoid and anaphylaxis, and (3) OPV and poliomyelitis.

[6]Infantile spasms and SIDS occur only in an age-group that is administered DT but not Td or tetanus toxoid.

[7]The evidence derived primarily from studies of DTP, although the evidence also favored rejection of a causal relationship between DT and SIDS.

[8]The evidence derived from studies of DT. If the evidence favored rejection of a causal relationship between DT and encephalopathy, then the evidence also favored rejection of a causal relationship between Td and tetanus toxoid and encephalopathy.

[9]The evidence derived from studies of tetanus toxoid. If the evidence favored acceptance of (or established) a causal relationship between tetanus toxoid and an adverse event, then the evidence also favored acceptance of (or established) a causal relationship between DT and Td and the adverse event.

[10]This conclusion differs from the information contained in the ACIP recommendations because of new information that became available after IOM published this table.

[11]Deaths occurred primarily among persons known to be immunocompromised.

Prophylaxis

Immune Globulin Preparations Available in the United States

Name	Manufacturer	Preparation	Dose Form	Plasma Source
Intramuscular Immune Globulin Preparations				
Generic	Massachusetts PHBL Michigan BPI New York Blood Center	Cold-ethanol fractionation, solvent-detergent treatment[1]	Solution (15%–18%)	Volunteer donors
Gammar-P IM	Centeon	Cold-ethanol fractionation, pasteurization at 60°C for 10 hours[1]	Solution (16.5±1%)	Paid donors
Intravenous Immune Globulin Preparations (Unselected)				
Venoglobulin-I	Alpha Therapeutic	PEG fractionation, DEAE-Sephadex ion-exchange adsorption	Lyophilized (5%)	Paid donors
Venoglobulin-S	Alpha Therapeutic	PEG fractionation, DEAE-Sephadex ion-exchange adsorption, solvent-detergent treatment	Solution (5% or 10%)	Paid donors
Polygam S/D	American Red Cross	pH 8, DEAE-Sephadex ion-exchange adsorption, solvent-detergent treatment	Lyophilized (5%)	Volunteer donors
Gammagard S/D	Baxter	pH 8, DEAE-Sephadex ion-exchange adsorption, solvent-detergent treatment	Lyophilized (5% or 10%)	Paid donors

Gamimune N	Bayer	Diafiltration and ultrafiltration	Solution (5% or 10%)	Paid donors
Gamimune N, Solvent/ Detergent Treated	Bayer	Limited diafiltration and ultrafiltration, solvent-detergent treatment, pH 4.25 at low salt at 20°C for 21 days	Solution (5% or 10%)	Paid donors
Gammar-P IV	Centeon	pH 7, ultrafiltration, pasteurization at 60°C for 10 hours	Lyophilized (5%)	Paid donors
Iveegam	Immuno AG	Trypsin treatment, isoelectric precipitation, PEG precipitation	Lyophilized (4.5%–5.5%)	Paid donors
Sandoglobulin	Novartis	pH 4.0 and pepsin treatment	Lyophilized (3%, 6%, 9%, or 12%)	Volunteer donors
Intravenous Immune Globulin Preparations, Hyperimmune[2]				
Cytomegalovirus immune globulin				
Cytogam	Massachusetts PHBL/ MedImmune[3]	Cold-ethanol fractionation, solvent-detergent treatment	Solution (4%–6%)	Paid and volunteer donors; selected plasma with high antibody titers to cytomegalovirus
Hepatitis B immune globulin (HBIG)				
H-BIG	Abbott/North American Biologicals[3]	Cold-ethanol fractionation	Solution (15%–18%)	Individuals hyperimmunized with hepatitis B vaccine
BayHep B	Bayer	Cold-ethanol fractionation, solvent-detergent treatment	Solution (15%–18%)	Paid donors

Table continued on following page

Name	Manufacturer	Preparation	Dose Form	Plasma Source
Human rabies immune globulin (HRIG)				
BayRab	Bayer	Cold-ethanol fractionation, solvent-detergent treatment	Solution (10%–18%)	Paid donors
Imogam Rabies-HT	Pasteur Mérieux Connaught[3]	Cold-ethanol fractionation, heat treatment	Solution (10%–18%)	Individuals hyperimmunized with rabies vaccine (HDCV)
Respiratory syncytial virus immune globulin, intravenous (RSV IGIV)				
RespiGam	Massachusetts PHBL/ MedImmune[3]	Cold-ethanol fractionation, ultrafiltration, solvent-detergent treatment	Solution (4%–6%)	Paid donors; selected plasma with high antibody titers to RSV
Tetanus immune globulin (TIG)				
BayTet	Bayer	Cold-ethanol fractionation, solvent-detergent treatment	Solution (15%–18%)	Individuals immunized with tetanus toxoid
Varicella-zoster virus immune globulin (VZIG)				
Varicella-zoster immune globulin	Massachusetts PHBL/ MedImmune[3]	Cold-ethanol fractionation, solvent-detergent treatment	Solution (10%–18%)	Volunteer donors; selected plasma with high antibody titers to VZV

[1]Unlike the processes used for IVIG, the process used for intramuscular immune globulin does not remove IgG aggregates.

[2]Pertussis immune globulin (PIG) was tried for treatment of pertussis but was not effective and is no longer available. Vaccinia immune globulin (VIG) was used for treatment of eczema vaccinatum, vaccinia necrosum, and ocular vaccinia. With the eradication of smallpox and discontinuation of smallpox vaccination, VIG is no longer available.

[3]Manufacturer/distributor(s).

Intramuscular Immune Globulin (IG)[1]

Indications

- Preexposure prophylaxis
  - Hepatitis A
    - Short term (1–2 months): 0.02 mL/kg
    - Long term (3–5 months): 0.06 mL/kg, and repeated every 5 months while continued exposure to hepatitis A virus occurs
- Postexposure prophylaxis
  - Hepatitis A: IG, 0.02 mL/kg, as soon as possible but not >2 weeks after exposure; if hepatitis A vaccine is recommended for the person receiving IG, vaccine may be administered simultaneously with IG but at a separate anatomical site (page 164)
  - Measles (page 178)
    - Normal contacts: IG, 0.25 mL/kg (maximum dose 15 mL), as soon as possible after exposure for susceptible household and hospital contacts, especially infants <6 months of age born to nonimmune mothers, infants 6–12 months of age, and pregnant women
    - Immunocompromised contacts (including persons with symptomatic HIV infection): IG, 0.5 mL/kg (maximum dose 15 mL), regardless of immunization status

Precautions

- Persons with a history of systemic allergic reactions following administration of human IG products
- Immunization with MMR live-virus vaccine should be deferred for 3 months (for 0.02 mL/kg or 0.06 mL/kg), 5 months (for 0.25 mL/kg), or 6 months (for 0.5 mL/kg) after IG administration (page 112)
- Immunization with varicella live-virus vaccine should be deferred for 5 months (for 0.02 mL/kg, 0.06 mL/kg, or 0.25 mL/kg) or 6 months (for 0.5 mL/kg) after IG administration (page 112)

---

[1]Formerly known as immune serum globulin (ISG).

Administration

- By intramuscular injection into the deltoid or gluteal muscle (or the anterolateral aspect of the mid-thigh for children <24 months of age)

Intravenous Immune Globulin (IVIG)

Indications[1]

- Immune globulin replacement therapy for antibody deficiency states
- Prevention of bacterial infections in patients with chronic lymphocytic leukemia
- Prevention of bacterial infections and graft-versus-host disease in bone marrow transplant patients >20 years of age during the first 100 days after transplant
- Prevention of bacterial infections in children with congenital or acquired immunodeficiency diseases, including HIV infection, who have recurrent, serious bacterial infections (i.e., ≥2 episodes in a 1-year period of bacteremia, meningitis, or pneumonia); data are inadequate to evaluate similar use in HIV-infected adults
- Treatment of immune thrombocytopenic purpura (ITP)
- Treatment of Kawasaki syndrome

Possible Indication

- As adjunctive therapy for treatment of neonatal sepsis

Precautions

- Persons with a history of systemic allergic reactions following administration of human immune globulin products
- Immunization with live-virus vaccines (e.g., MMR, varicella) should be deferred for 5 months (for 400 mg/kg), 6 months (for 1000 mg/kg), or 11 months (for 2000 mg/kg) after IVIG administration (page 112)

Administration

- By intravenous administration

---

[1]Additional off-label indications for IVIG use are found in ASHP Commission on Therapeutics. ASHP therapeutic guidelines for intravenous immune globulin. *Clin Pharm* 1992;11:117–136; Ratko TA, Burnett DA, Foulke GE, et al. Recommendations for off-label use of intravenously administered immunoglobulin preparations. *JAMA* 1995;273:1865–1870.

Cytomegalovirus Intravenous Immune Globulin (CMV IVIG)

Indications

- Prophylaxis of CMV disease associated with kidney transplantation, especially in CMV-seronegative recipients from CMV-seropositive donors[1]
- Treatment (with ganciclovir) of CMV disease (e.g., pneumonia) associated with bone marrow and solid organ transplantation

Possible Indication

- Prophylaxis of CMV disease associated with bone marrow and solid organ transplantation, especially in CMV-seronegative recipients from CMV-seropositive donors[1]

Precautions

- Persons with a history of systemic allergic reactions following administration of human immune globulin products
- Immunization with live-virus vaccines (e.g., MMR, varicella) should be deferred for 5–9 months after CMV IVIG administration[2]

Administration

- *Prophylaxis:* 500 mg/kg weekly for 90 days[1]
- *Treatment:* ganciclovir, 7.5 mg/kg/day intravenously divided every 8 hours for 14 days with CMV IVIG, 400 mg/kg on days 1, 2, and 7, and 200 mg/kg on day 14[3]

---

[1]A uniform prophylaxis regimen for CMV infection has not been developed. Both CMV IVIG and IVIG reduce the incidence of CMV disease in patients receiving transplantations.

[2]There are no specific published recommended intervals between administration of CMV IVIG and vaccination with preparations containing live virus (measles/MMR or varicella) (page 112).

[3]Reed EC, Bowden RA, Dandliker PS, et al. Treatment of cytomegalovirus pneumonia with ganciclovir and intravenous cytomegalovirus immunoglobulin in patients with bone marrow transplants. *Ann Intern Med* 1988;109:783–788.

- *Alternative regimen using IVIG:* ganciclovir, 7.5 mg/kg/day intravenously divided every 8 hours for 20 days with IVIG, 500 mg/kg every other day for 10 doses[4]

[4] Emanuel D, Cunningham I, Jules-Elysee K, et al. Cytomegalovirus pneumonia after bone marrow transplantation successfully treated with the combination of ganciclovir and high-dose intravenous immune globulin. *Ann Intern Med* 1988; 109:772–782.

Hepatitis B Immune Globulin (HBIG)

Indications

- Postexposure prophylaxis
  - Sexual exposure (acute case of chronic HBsAg carrier)
  - Household exposure to acute case
  - Household exposure to chronic HBsAg carrier
  - Percutaneous or permucosal exposure
- Perinatal exposure (infant born to a mother who is HbsAg positive)

Precautions

- Persons with a history of systemic allergic reactions following administration of human immune globulin products
- Immunization with live-virus vaccines should be deferred for 3 months (MMR) or 5 months (varicella) after HBIG administration

Administration

- Postexposure prophylaxis (page 166)
  - 0.06 mL/kg intramuscularly as soon as possible after exposure and initiation or completion of hepatitis B vaccine series (A second dose of HBIG should be administered 1 month later if the hepatitis B vaccine series has not been started.)
- Prenatal exposure (page 205)
  - HBIG, 0.5 mL intramuscularly within 12 hours of birth
  - Hepatitis B vaccine (first dose), 0.5 mL intramuscularly within 12 hours of birth

Human Rabies Immune Globulin (HRIG)

Indication

- Postexposure prophylaxis for prevention of rabies, up to 8 days after the first vaccine dose (page 183)

Contraindication

- Persons who have been completely immunized with rabies vaccine and are known to have an adequate antibody titer

Precautions

- Persons with a history of systemic allergic reactions following administration of human immune globulin products
- Immunization with live-virus vaccines should be deferred for 4 months (for MMR) or 5 months (for varicella) after HRIG administration

Administration

- *After immediate thorough cleansing of all bite wounds and scratches with soap and water:*
  - HRIG, 20 IU/kg (0.133 mL/kg) as soon as possible, with the first dose of rabies vaccine, if anatomically feasible, the full dose of HRIG should be thoroughly infiltrated in the area around and into the wound(s); if not anatomically feasible, any remaining volume should be administered intramuscularly at a site distant from vaccine inoculation

Respiratory Syncytial Virus Immune Globulin, Intravenous (RSV IGIV)

Indications

- Infants and children younger than 2 years of age with bronchopulmonary dysplasia who are currently receiving or have received oxygen therapy within the 6 months before the anticipated RSV season
  - Severe lung disease: prophylaxis for first two RSV seasons
  - Less severe lung disease: first-season RSV only
- Infants with a gestational age of ≤32 weeks without bronchopulmonary dysplasia
  - Gestational age of ≤28 weeks: prophylaxis up to 12 months of age
  - Gestational age of 29–32 weeks: prophylaxis up to 6 months of age

Possible Indication

- Children with severe immunodeficiencies (e.g., severe combined immunodeficiency or severe acquired immunodeficiency syndrome) receiving monthly IVIG infusions may benefit from substituting RSV IGIV during the RSV season

Contraindication

- Patients with cyanotic chronic heart disease without bronchopulmonary dysplasia or not born prematurely

Precautions

- Persons with a history of systemic allergic reactions following administration of human immune globulin products
- Immunization with live virus vaccines (e.g., MMR, varicella) should be deferred for 9 months after RSV IGIV administration

Not a Contraindication

- Patients with asymptomatic acyanotic chronic heart disease (e.g., patent ductus arteriosus or ventricular septal defect)

Administration

- RSV IGIV, 750 mg/kg/dose monthly at the beginning of the RSV season (October to December) and terminated at the end of the RSV season (March to May)[1]

[1]Regional and annual differences occur; the onset of RSV occurs earlier in southern states than in northern states; in most areas of the United States, RSV season begins in October to December and subsides in March to May.

Tetanus Immune Globulin (TIG)

Indications

- Prophylaxis (e.g., for wound management)
  - Individuals with uncertain tetanus immunization history or <3 immunizations with wounds contaminated with dirt, feces, and saliva; puncture wounds; avulsions; and wounds resulting from missiles, crushing, burns, and frostbite (page 186)
  - HIV-1–infected individuals with wounds contaminated with dirt, feces, and saliva; puncture wounds; avulsions; and wounds resulting from missiles, crushing, burns, and frostbite (regardless of the history of tetanus immunizations)
- Treatment of tetanus

Precautions

- Persons with a history of systemic allergic reactions following administration of human immune globulin products
- Immunization with live-virus vaccines should be deferred for 3 months (for MMR) or 5 months (for varicella) after TIG administration

Administration

- Prophylaxis (e.g., for wound management; with tetanus vaccine administration)
  - Clean, minor wounds: 250 units (1 mL) intramuscularly into the gluteal muscle
  - Severe wounds, tetanus-prone wounds, or delay in treatment: 500 units (2 mL) intramuscularly into the gluteal muscle; the prophylaxis dosage may be increased to 1000–2000 units
- Treatment of tetanus (with antibiotics and appropriate supportive care): 3000–6000 units intramuscularly into the gluteal muscle; a portion of the dose may be administered around the wound, although the efficacy of this approach has not been proven

Varicella-Zoster Immune Globulin (VZIG)

Indications

- *Perinatal exposure*
  - Newborn infant of a mother with onset of maternal rash of chickenpox within 5 days before delivery to within 48 hours after delivery
- *Other exposure*
  - Susceptible individuals who have close and prolonged exposure to a case or to an infectious hospital staff worker or patient
    - Immunocompromised children <15 years of age without a history of chickenpox
    - Immunocompromised adolescents and adults ≥15 years of age with known susceptibility
    - Immunocompetent adolescents and adults ≥15 years of age with known susceptibility
    - Pregnant women with no history of chickenpox
    - Premature infants ≥28 weeks' gestation and <40 weeks postconceptional age whose mothers have no history of chickenpox
    - Premature infants <28 weeks' gestation or birth weight ≤1000 g, and <40 weeks after conceptional age, regardless of maternal history of chickenpox

and

- Significant exposure to a person with chickenpox or zoster
  - Continuous household contact
  - Playmate contact (more than 1 hour of indoor play)
  - Hospital contact
    - In the same 2- to 4-bedroom, or
    - In adjacent beds in large wards, or
    - Having prolonged face-to-face contact with an infectious employee or staff member, household member, or patient

and

- The time elapsed permits administration of VZIG within 96 hours of exposure (given as soon as possible)

Precautions

- Persons with a history of systemic allergic reactions following administration of human immune globulin products
- Immunization with live-virus vaccines (e.g., MMR, varicella) should be deferred for 5 months after VZIG administration

Administration

- VZIG, 125 units (minimum dose) for each 10-kg increment of body weight to a maximum dose of 625 units intramuscularly into the gluteal muscle

Postexposure Prophylaxis

Cholera

Indication

- Selective chemoprophylaxis administered within 24 hours for members of a household who share food and shelter with a cholera patient in communities with a high secondary attack rate (at least one household member in five becomes ill after the 1st case occurs in a household)
  - Not usually necessary in the United States unless poor sanitary and hygiene conditions indicate the likelihood of secondary transmission
  - Mass chemoprophylaxis is ineffective, diverts attention and resources, and contributes to emergence of resistance

Recommended Regimens[1,2]

Age-Group	Antibiotic
Adults ≥18 years	Doxycycline,[1] 300 mg orally as a single dose, *or* Tetracycline, 500 mg orally 4 times per day for 3 days, *or* Ciprofloxacin, 500 mg orally twice per day for 3 days, *or* Co-trimoxazole, TMP, 160 mg, with SMX, 800 mg, orally twice per day for 3 days, *or* Furazolidone,[3] 100 mg orally 4 times per day for 3 days

[1]Doxycycline is the antibiotic of choice (except for children <9 years of age and pregnant women) because only 1 dose is required. A single dose of doxycycline is probably safe for children <9 years of age.

[2]Erythromycin or chloramphenicol may be used if these antibiotics are not available or where *Vibrio cholerae* O1 is resistant to these antibiotics.

[3]Furazolidone is the antibiotic of choice for pregnant women.

Table continued on following page

Age-Group	Antibiotic
Children ≥9 years	Doxycycline,[1] 6 mg/kg orally as a single dose, *or* Tetracycline, 50 mg/kg/day orally divided 4 times per day for 3 days, *or* Co-trimoxazole, TMP, 10 mg/kg/day, with SMX, 50 mg/kg/day, orally divided twice per day for 3 days, *or* Furazolidone, 5 mg/kg/day orally divided 4 times per day for 3 days
Children ≥2 months[4]	Co-trimoxazole, TMP, 5 mg/kg/day, with SMX, 25 mg/kg/day, orally divided twice per day for 3 days

[4]Co-trimoxazole is the antibiotic of choice for children. A single dose of doxycycline is probably safe for children <9 years of age.

Pharyngeal Diphtheria (*Corynebacterium diphtheriae*)[1]

Indication

- Persons with close exposure to persons suspected or proved to have pharyngeal diphtheria

Recommended Regimens

- Chemoprophylaxis
  - Erythromycin, 40–50 mg/kg/day (maximum daily dose, 2g/day) orally divided every 6 hours for 7 days, *or*
  - Benzathine penicillin G, 600,000–1,200,000 units intramuscularly as a single dose[2]

and

- Vaccination with DPT, DT, or Td (depending on age) for the following groups:
  - Unimmunized persons
  - Previously immunized close contacts who have not received a booster dose of diphtheria toxoid within 5 years
  - Persons for whom the immunization status is not known

[1]All close contacts should also have a nasopharyngeal culture for *C. diphtheriae* and should be observed for 7 days for evidence of disease.

[2]Recommended for persons who cannot be kept under surveillance.

Haemophilus influenzae type b

HIGH-RISK CONTACTS AND INDEX CASES OF PATIENTS WITH INVASIVE INFECTION

Household Exposure

- Indications
  - Households with at least 1 contact[1] younger than 48 months of age who did not have at least 1 dose of conjugate vaccine at ≥15 months of age, 2 doses between 12 and 14 months of age, or a 2- or 3-dose primary series when younger than 12 months of age with a booster dose at ≥12 months of age
  - Households with an immunocompromised child, regardless of immunization status or age
- Recipients
  - All household contacts should receive rifampin as soon as possible; prophylaxis ≥7 days after hospitalization of the index patient, although not optimal, may still provide benefit
  - The index case of households receiving prophylaxis should receive rifampin prophylaxis if treated with ampicillin or chloramphenicol; if treatment was with cefotaxime or ceftriaxone, prophylaxis of the index case is not necessary since these drugs, in contrast to ampicillin and chloramphenicol, eradicate *H. influenzae* type b from the nasopharynx

Childcare and Nursery School Exposure

- Indications
  - Two or more cases of invasive Hib disease within 60 days *and* attendees include children with incomplete Hib vaccination

[1]A household contact is defined as an individual residing with the index patient or a nonresident who spent ≥4 hours with the index patient for at least 5 of the 7 days preceding the day of hospital admission of the index patient.

- A single case of invasive Hib disease *and* attendees include unvaccinated or incompletely vaccinated children <2 years of age *and* contact is ≥25 hours/week

- Recipients
  - All attendees and supervisory personnel should receive rifampin as soon as possible; prophylaxis ≥7 days after hospitalization of the index patient, although not optimal, may still provide benefit
  - The index case of groups receiving prophylaxis should receive rifampin prophylaxis if treated with ampicillin or chloramphenicol; if treatment was with cefotaxime or ceftriaxone, prophylaxis of the index case is not necessary since these drugs, in contrast to ampicillin and chloramphenicol, eradicate *H. influenzae* type b from the nasopharynx

Recommended Regimens

- Rifampin: for household exposure, all household contacts of the unvaccinated or incompletely vaccinated children should receive chemoprophylaxis with rifampin
  - <1 month of age: 10 mg/kg orally every 24 hours for 4 days
  - 1 month to 12 years of age: 20 mg/kg orally every 24 hours for 4 days
  - >12 years of age (adults): 600 mg every 24 hours for 4 days
- Hib vaccination: unvaccinated or incompletely vaccinated children should receive 1 dose of vaccine and should be scheduled for completion of the age-specific immunization schedule (page 54)

Hepatitis A

Indications for Immune Globulin Prophylaxis (within 2 Weeks of Exposure)

- Household and sexual contacts of persons with serologically confirmed hepatitis A and who have not been vaccinated ≥1 month before exposure
- Staff and attendees of day care centers or homes
  - With 1 or more cases of hepatitis A in employees or attendees
  - With cases in 2 or more households of center attendees; in centers that do not provide care to children who wear diapers, IG need be given only to classroom contacts of an index case
- Members of households of day care center attendees in diapers when hepatitis A occurs in three or more families
- Common-source exposure from a food handler
  - For other food handlers at the same location (also consider administration of hepatitis A vaccine)
  - For patrons if (1) during the time when the food handler was likely to be infectious the food handler handled uncooked foods or foods after cooking and had diarrhea or poor hygienic practices and (2) patrons can be identified and treated within 2 weeks after the exposure
  - Close contacts only if an epidemiological investigation indicates hepatitis A virus transmission among students in a school or among patients or between patients and staff in a hospital

Not Indications

- Contacts of a single case in an elementary or secondary school, an office, or other work setting
- Health-care workers for a patient with hepatitis A

Special Considerations

- IG may interfere with live virus vaccines. Administration of MMR vaccines should be delayed for at least 3 months, and varicella vaccine should be delayed for at least 5 months, after administration of IG for hepatitis A postexposure prophylaxis (page 112). IG does not interfere with the immune response to oral poliovirus vaccine or yellow fever vaccine, or, in general, to inactivated vaccines.

- If IG is administered within 2 weeks after administration of measles, mumps, or rubella vaccines or within 3 weeks after administration of varicella vaccine, the person should be revaccinated, but not sooner than 3 months after IG administration for MMR or 5 months for varicella vaccine (page 111).
- Preexposure prophylaxis using hepatitis A vaccine is indicated for populations at increased risk and for certain international travelers ≥2 years of age if given >14 days prior to travel, or with IG if exposure will occur within 14 days (page 76). Preexposure prophylaxis using IG alone is indicated for certain international travelers <2 years of age (page 258).

Recommended Regimens

Age of Person Exposed	Time Since Last Exposure	Likelihood of Future Exposure	Postexposure Prophylaxis[1,2]
<2 years	<2 weeks	Unlikely	IG (0.02 mL/kg)
		Likely	IG (0.02 mL/kg)
	>2 weeks	Unlikely	No postexposure prophylaxis
		Likely	IG (0.02 mL/kg)
≥2 years	<2 weeks	Unlikely	IG (0.02 mL/kg)
		Likely	IG (0.02 mL/kg) and hepatitis A vaccine series (page 76)
	>2 weeks	Unlikely	No postexposure prophylaxis
		Likely	Hepatitis A vaccine series (page 76)

[1]IG postexposure prophylaxis should be given as soon as possible but not >2 weeks after the last exposure. If future exposure is likely, hepatitis A vaccine and IG may be administered simultaneously at separate anatomical sites.

[2]Persons who have received one dose of hepatitis A vaccine ≥1 month before exposure to hepatitis A do not need to receive IG.

Hepatitis B

Perinatal Exposure (page 205)

- Indication: infants born to HBsAg-positive mothers
- Regimen
  - HBIG, 0.5 mL intramuscularly within 12 hours of birth
  - Hepatitis B vaccine (first dose), 0.5 mL intramuscularly within 12 hours of birth (and then complete the series)

Sexual Exposure (Acute Case or Chronic HBsAg Carrier)

- Indications
  - Sexual partners of persons with acute hepatitis B infection within 14 days of last sexual contact *or* if sexual contact will continue
  - Sexual partners of chronic HBsAg-positive persons
- Regimen
  - HBIG, 0.06 mL/kg intramuscularly
  - Hepatitis B vaccination (first dose immediately and then complete the series)

Household Exposure to Acute Case of Hepatitis B

- Indications
  - Infant <12 months of age not previously vaccinated against hepatitis B
  - Household contact with identifiable blood exposure to the index patient (e.g., by sharing toothbrushes or razors)
- Regimen
  - HBIG, 0.06 mL/kg intramuscularly
  - Hepatitis B vaccination (first dose immediately and then complete the series)

Household Exposure to Chronic HBsAg Carrier

- Indications: all household contacts
- Regimen: hepatitis B vaccination

Percutaneous or Permucosal Exposure

	Treatment When Source Patient is Found to Be:		
Exposed Person	**HBsAg Positive**	**HBsAg Negative**	**Source Patient Not Tested or Unknown**
Unvaccinated	HBIG (at exposure)[1] and initiate hepatitis B vaccine series[2]	Initiate hepatitis B vaccine series[2]	Initiate hepatitis B vaccine series[2]
Previously Vaccinated			
Known responder[3]	No treatment	No treatment	No treatment
Known nonresponder	HBIG (at exposure and repeated at 1 month) *or* HBIG (at exposure) and hepatitis B vaccine booster dose	No treatment	If known high-risk source, treat as if source were HbsAg positive
Response unknown	Test exposed person for anti-HBs[4]: If adequate,[3] no treatment If inadequate,[3] HBIG (at exposure) and hepatitis B vaccine booster dose	No treatment	Test exposed person for anti-HBs[4]: If adequate,[3] no treatment If inadequate,[3] hepatitis B vaccine booster dose

Table continued on following page

Adapted from Centers for Disease Control and Prevention: Protection against viral hepatitis: recommendations of the Immunization Practices Advisory Committee (ACIP). *MMWR Morb Mortal Wkly Rep* 1990;39(RR-2):15–16.

[1]HBIG, 0.06 mL/kg intramuscularly, should be administered as soon as possible, preferably within 24 hours but at least within 7 days.

[2]See page 59 for hepatitis B vaccine dosages and schedules.

[3]A responder is defined as a person with adequate levels of serum antibody to hepatitis B surface antigen (i.e., hepatitis B surface antibody [anti-HBs] ≥10 mIU/mL by RIA or EIA); inadequate response to vaccination is defined as serum anti-HBs <10 mIU/mL.

[4]It is not necessary to test for anti-HBs if the exposed person has been tested within the past 24 months and an adequate level has been demonstrated.

Hepatitis C

Postexposure Prophylaxis

- Currently there is no recommended postexposure prophylaxis regimen for hepatitis C virus (HCV); use of immune globulin is not recommended since all blood is now screened for anti-HCV and is not used if positive for anti-HCV

Postexposure Management[1]

- Baseline serology for anti-HCV; if positive, the HCV infection is not related to that exposure
- HCV PCR at 2–3 weeks, and repeat anti-HCV at 6 weeks, 3 months, and 6 months; persons with a positive PCR or seroconversion should be referred to a hepatologist for evaluation for early α-interferon therapy; persons with negative anti-HCV tests require no further evaluation

---

Adapted from Centers for Disease Control and Prevention. Immunization of health-care workers: recommendations of the Advisory Committee on Immunization Practices (ACIP) and the Hospital Infection Control Practices Advisory Committee (HICPAC). *MMWR Morb Mortal Wkly Rep* 1997;46(RR-18): 14–17, 26.

[1]The CDC guidelines state that institutions may "consider" follow-up testing but do not specifically recommend HCV PCR testing. Many experts recommend early testing for HCV PCR to facilitate earlier diagnosis than would be possible by anti-HCV antibody testing, which could allow for earlier therapy and thus possibly a greater chance of preventing disease.

Human Immunodeficiency Virus (HIV)

STEP 1: Determine the Exposure Code (EC)

Is the source material blood, bloody fluid, other potentially infectious material (OPIM),[1] or an instrument contaminated with one of these substances?

- Yes
  - OPIM[2]
  - Blood or bloody fluid
- No → No PEP needed

What type of exposure has occurred?

- Mucous membrane or skin integrity compromised[3] → Volume
  - **Small** (e.g., few drops, short duration) → EC 1
  - **Large** (e.g., several drops, major blood splash, and/or longer duration [i.e., several minutes or more]) → EC 2
- Intact skin only[4] → No PEP needed
- Percutaneous exposure → Severity
  - **Less Severe** (e.g., solid needle, superficial scratch) → EC 2
  - **More Severe** (e.g., large-bore hollow needle, deep puncture, visible blood on device, or needle used in source patient's artery or vein)[5] → EC 3

[1]Semen or vaginal secretions; cerebrospinal, synovial, pleural, peritoneal, pericardial, or amniotic fluids; or tissue.

[2]Exposures to OPIM must be evaluated on a case-by-case basis. In general, these body substances are considered a low risk for transmission in health-care settings. Any unprotected contact to concentrated HIV in a research laboratory or production facility is considered an occupational exposure that requires clinical evaluation to determine the need for PEP.

[3]Skin integrity is considered compromised if there is evidence of chapped skin, dermatitis, abrasion, or open wound.

[4]Contact with intact skin is not normally considered a risk for HIV transmission. However, if the exposure was to blood and the circumstance suggests a higher volume exposure (e.g., an extensive area of skin was exposed or there was prolonged contact with blood), the risk for HIV transmission should be considered.

[5]The combination of these severity factors (e.g., large-bore hollow needle *and* deep puncture) contributes to an elevated risk for transmission if the source person is HIV-positive.

STEP 2: Determine the HIV Status Code (HIV SC)

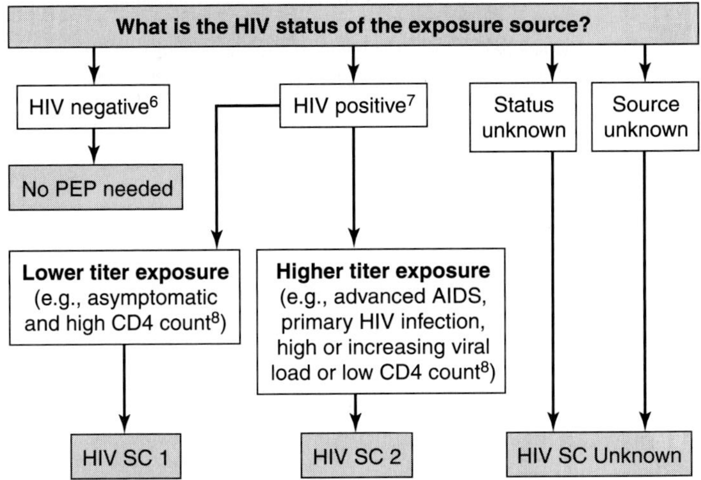

[6]A source is considered negative for HIV infection if there is laboratory documentation of a negative HIV antibody, HIV polymerase chain reaction (PCR), or HIV p24 antigen test result from a specimen collected at or near the time of exposure and there is no clinical evidence of recent retroviral-like illness.

[7]A source is considered infected with HIV (HIV positive) if there has been a positive laboratory result for HIV antibody, HIV PCR, or HIV p24 antigen or physician-diagnosed AIDS.

[8]Examples are used as surrogates to estimate the HIV titer in an exposure source for purposes of considering PEP regimens and do not reflect all clinical situations that may be observed. Although a high HIV titer (HIV SC 2) in an exposure source has been associated with an increased risk for transmission, the possibility of transmission from a source with a low HIV titer also must be considered.

STEP 3: Determine the PEP Recommendation

EC	HIV SC	PEP Recommendation
1	1	**PEP may not be warrented.** Exposure type does not pose a known risk for HIV transmission. Whether the risk for drug toxicity outweighs the benefit of PEP should be decided by the exposed HCW and treating clinician.
1	2	**Consider basic regimen.**[9] Exposure type poses a negligible risk for HIV transmission. A high HIV titer in the source may justify consideration of PEP. Whether the risk for drug toxicity outweighs the benefit of PEP should be decided by the exposed HCW and treating clinician.
2	1	**Recommend basic regimen.** Most HIV exposures are in this category; no increased risk for HIV transmission has been observed but use of PEP is appropriate.
2	2	**Recommend expanded regimen.**[10] Exposure type represents an increased HIV transmission risk.
3	1 or 2	**Recommend expanded regimen.** Exposure type represents an increased HIV transmission risk.
Unknown		If the source or, in the case of an unknown source, the setting where the exposure occurred suggests a possible risk for HIV exposure and the EC is 2 or 3, consider PEP basic regimen.

[9]Basic regimen is four weeks of zidovudine, 600 mg per day in two or three divided doses, *and* lamivudine, 150 mg twice daily (page 173).
[10]Expanded regimen is the basic regimen plus *either* indinavir, 800 mg every 8 hours, *or* nelfinavir, 750 mg three times a day (page 173).

Adapted from Centers for Disease Control and Prevention. Public Health Service guidelines for the management of health-care worker exposures to HIV and recommendations for postexposure prophylaxis. *MMWR Morb Mortal Wkly Rep* 1998;47(RR-7):14–15. This algorithm is intended to guide initial decisions about postexposure prophylaxis (PEP) and should be used in conjunction with other guidance provided by a specialist, or in this report.

Basic and Expanded HIV Postexposure Prophylaxis Regimens

Regimen Category	Application	Drug Regimen
Basic	Occupational HIV exposures for which there is a recognized transmission risk (Figure, pages 170–172)	4 weeks (28 days) of both zidovudine 600 mg every day in divided doses (i.e., 300 mg twice a day, 200 mg three times per day, or 100 mg every 4 hours) *and* lamivudine 150 mg twice a day
Expanded	Occupational HIV exposures that pose an increased risk for transmission (e.g., larger volume of blood and/or higher virus titer in blood [Figure, pages 170–172])	Basic regimen plus *either* indinavir 800 mg every 8 hours *or* nelfinavir 750 mg three times a day[1]

Adapted from Centers for Disease Control and Prevention. Public Health Service guidelines for the management of health-care worker exposures to HIV and recommendations for postexposure prophylaxis. *MMWR Morb Mortal Wkly Rep* 1988;47(RR-7):21.

[1]Indinavir should be taken on an empty stomach (i.e., without food or with a light meal) and with increased fluid consumption (i.e., drinking six 8 oz glasses of water throughout the day); nelfinavir should be taken with meals.

HIV Postexposure Prophylaxis Resources and Registries

Resource or Registry	Contact Information	
National Clinician's Postexposure Hotline	Telephone:	888-448-4911
HIV Postexposure Prophylaxis Registry	Telephone:	888-737-4448 (888-PEP4HIV)
	Address:	1410 Commonwealth Drive Suite 215 Wilmington, NC 28405
Antiretroviral Pregnancy Registry	Telephone:	800-258-4263
	Fax:	800-800-1052
	Address:	1410 Commonwealth Drive Suite 215 Wilmington, NC 28405
Food and Drug Administration (for reporting unusual or severe toxicity to antiretroviral agents)	Telephone:	800-332-1088
CDC (for reporting HIV seroconversion in health-care workers who received postexposure prophylaxis)	Telephone:	404-639-6425

Influenza

Indications

- Persons who receive influenza vaccination at a time when influenza A is already present in the community (continue chemoprophylaxis for 2 weeks after vaccination; in children receiving initial influenza vaccination, for 2 weeks after the second dose of vaccine [6 weeks total])
- During the period of peak influenza A activity
  - Persons who cannot be vaccinated
  - Persons with immunodeficiency (including HIV infection) who are expected to have an inadequate response to influenza vaccine
- During community *influenza A* outbreaks
  - Unvaccinated persons who have frequent contact with persons at high risk (e.g., household members, visiting nurses, volunteer workers)
  - Unvaccinated health-care workers of hospitals, clinics, and chronic-care facilities
  - Chemoprophylaxis should be considered for vaccinated and unvaccinated nonill health-care workers in closed or semiclosed settings (e.g., hospitals, clinics, chronic care facilities) where persons at risk for influenza-related complications are in close proximity if the outbreak is caused by a variant strain of influenza A that might not be controlled by the vaccine[2]

Adapted from Centers for Disease Control and Prevention. Prevention and control of influenza: recommendations of the Advisory Committee on Immunization Practices (ACIP). *MMWR Morb Mortal Wkly Rep* 1998;47(RR-6):18.

[1]Chemoprophylaxis is not a substitute for influenza vaccination. When feasible, measures should be taken to reduce the contact between symptomatic and asymptomatic persons during outbreaks.

[2]These antiviral drugs can also be used to reduce the severity and duration of influenza A illness when treatment is initiated within 48 hours of illness onset.

- During influenza A outbreaks in closed or semiclosed settings where persons at risk for influenza-related complications are in close proximity (continue chemoprophylaxis for at least 2 weeks, or 1 week after the end of the outbreak)
  - Vaccinated and unvaccinated residents of chronic-care facilities
  - Unvaccinated health-care workers who provide care to persons at high risk
- Any person who desires to avoid influenza illness

Recommended Regimens

Antiviral Agent	Age (Years) 1–9	10–13	14–64	≥65
Amantadine[1,2]				
Prophylaxis[3]	5 mg/kg/day (maximum daily dose, 150 mg) orally in 2 divided doses	100 mg orally twice daily[4]	100 mg orally twice daily	≤100 mg/day
Treatment	5 mg/kg/day (maximum daily dose, 150 mg) orally in 2 divided doses	100 mg orally twice daily[4]	100 mg orally twice daily	≤100 mg/day
Rimantadine[1,2]				
Prophylaxis[3]	5 mg/kg/day (maximum daily dose, 150 mg) orally in 2 divided doses	100 mg orally twice daily[4]	100 mg orally twice daily	100 or 200 mg/day[5]
Treatment	Not approved	Not approved	100 mg orally twice daily	100 or 200 mg/day[5]

Adapted from Centers for Disease Control and Prevention. Prevention and control of influenza: recommendations of the Advisory Committee on Immunization Practices (ACIP). *MMWR Morb Mortal Wkly Rep* 1998;47(RR-6):18.

[1]Amantadine manufacturers include DuPont Pharma (Symmetrel; syrup); Chase Pharmaceuticals, Invamed, and Endo Pharmaceuticals (Amantadine HCl; capsule); and Copley Pharmaceuticals, Barre National, and Mikart (Amantadine HCl; syrup). Rimantadine is manufactured by Forest Laboratories (Flumadine; tablet and syrup).

Table continued on following page

Dosage Adjustments for Renal Impairment

Amantadine

CrCl 30–50 mL/min/1.73 m^2	One-half the daily dose each day (100 mg/day for adults)
CrCl 15–29 mL/min/1.73 m^2	Usual daily dose on day 1; one-half the daily dose every other day thereafter (200 mg once, then 100 mg/day for adults)
CrCl <15 mL/min/1.73 m^2	Usual daily dose once every 7 days (200 mg/7 days for adults)

Rimantadine

CrCl ≤10 mL/min/1.73 m^2	One-half the usual daily dose (100 mg/day for adults)

Dosage Adjustments for Hepatic Impairment

Amantadine	No dosage reduction is necessary
Rimantadine	A reduction in dosage to 100 mg/day of rimantadine is recommended for persons who have severe hepatic dysfunction or those with creatinine clearance 10 mL/min/1.73 m^2. Other persons with less severe hepatic or renal dysfunction taking >100 mg/day of rimantadine should be observed closely, and the dosage should be reduced or the drug discontinued, if necessary.

[2]The package insert should be consulted for dosage recommendations for administering amantadine to persons with creatinine clearance ≤50 mL/min/1.73 m^2.

[3]To be maximally effective as prophylaxis, amantadine or rimantadine must be taken each day for the duration of influenza activity in the community. However, to be most cost-effective, prophylaxis should be taken only during the period of peak influenza activity in a community.

[4]Children ≥10 years of age who weigh <40 kg should be administered amantadine or rimantadine at a dose of 5 mg/kg/day.

[5]Elderly nursing-home residents should be given only 100 mg of rimandine per day. A reduction in dose to 100 mg/day should be considered for all persons ≥65 years of age if they experience side effects when taking 200 mg/day.

Measles

Indications

- Measles vaccine: infants and children ≥6 months of age who have not received measles vaccine
- Immune globulin: susceptible household and hospital contacts, especially infants <6 months of age born to nonimmune mothers, infants 6–12 months of age, pregnant women, and immunocompromised persons, including HIV-infected persons who are symptomatic or who are severely immunocompromised (page 39)

Recommended Regimens

Susceptible Individual	Measles Vaccine (Given within 72 Hours)	Immune Globulin (IG)[1,2] (Given within 6 Days)
≤6 months of age		
Mother is immune	No	No
Mother is nonimmune	No	0.25 mL/kg[3]
6–12 months of age	Yes	0.25 mL/kg[3]
≥12 months of age	Yes	No
Pregnant women	No	0.25 mL/kg[3]
Immunocompromised persons (including persons with symptomatic HIV infection) regardless of immunization status	No	0.5 mL/kg[3]

[1]IG postexposure prophylaxis should be given as soon as possible but not >6 days after the last exposure. If measles vaccine is recommended for the person receiving IG, they may be administered simultaneously at separate anatomical sites.

[2]Administration of live-virus vaccines is not recommended for at least 5 months following IG administration of 0.25 mL/kg or for at least 6 months following 0.5 mL/kg (page 112).

[3]Maximum dose 15 mL.

Meningococcus *(Neisseria meningitidis)*[1]

High-Risk Factors (Chemoprophylaxis Recommended)

- Household contacts, especially young children
- Childcare or nursery school contact in previous 7 days
- Direct exposure to the index patient's secretions through kissing or sharing toothbrushes or eating utensils
- Mouth-to-mouth resuscitation or unprotected contact during endotracheal intubation within 7 days before onset of illness
- Frequently sleeps or eats in the same dwelling as the index patient

Low-Risk Factors (Chemoprophylaxis Not Recommended)

- Casual contact with no history of direct exposure to the index patient's oral secretions (e.g., school or work mate indirect contact)
- Indirect contact (i.e., the only contact is with a high-risk contact, with no direct contact with the index patient)
- Medical personnel without direct exposure to the patient's oral secretions

Outbreak or Cluster

- Chemoprophylaxis for persons other than those at high risk should be given only after consultation with local/state public health authorities

---

Adapted from American Academy of Pediatrics, Committee on Infectious Diseases, and Canadian Paediatric Society, Infectious Diseases and Immunization Committee. Meningococcal disease prevention and control strategies for practice-based physicians. *Pediatrics* 1996;97:406. Reproduced by permission of *Pediatrics* vol 96, page 406, 1996.

[1]Nasopharyngeal aspirate or throat swab cultures are not useful in determining risk.

Regimens for High-Risk Contacts and Index Cases of Invasive Meningococcal Disease

Regimen and Age of Contact	Regimen	Efficacy
Recommended Regimens		
Rifampin[1]		72%–90%
≤1 month of age	5 mg/kg orally every 12 hours for 2 days	
1 month to 12 years of age	10 mg/kg (maximum dose 600 mg) orally every 12 hours for 2 days *or* 20 mg/kg (maximum dose 600 mg) orally every 24 hours for 4 days	
Adolescents and adults	600 mg orally every 12 hours for 2 days *or* 600 mg orally every 24 hours for 4 days	
or		
Ceftriaxone		97%
≤12 years	125 mg intramuscularly once	
>12 years	250 mg intramuscularly once	
or		
Ciprofloxacin (adults only)[2]	500 mg orally once	90%–95%
Alternative Regimen		
Sulfisoxazole (only if the isolate from the index case is known to be sulfa susceptible)		
<1 year	500 mg orally every 24 hours for 2 days	
1–12 years	500 mg orally every 12 hours for 2 days	
>12 years	1 g orally every 12 hours for 2 days	

Adapted from American Academy of Pediatrics, Committee on Infectious Diseases, and Canadian Paediatric Society, Infectious Diseases and Immunization Committee. Meningococcal disease prevention and control strategies for practice-based physicians. *Pediatrics* 1996;97:407. Reproduced by permission of *Pediatrics* vol 97, page 407, 1996.

[1]Rifampin is contraindicated for pregnant women.

[2]Ciprofloxacin and other quinolone antibiotics are contraindicated for pregnant and lactating women, children, and adolescents younger than 18 years.

Pertussis (*Bordetella pertussis*)

Indication

- All household contacts and other close contacts, such as those in child care, of a case of pertussis, regardless of age and vaccination status[1]

Recommended Regimen

Erythromycin 40–50 mg/kg/day (maximum daily dose, 2 g/day) orally divided in 4 daily doses for 14 days

Alternative Regimens[2]

Clarithromycin 15 mg/kg/day (maximum daily dose, 1 g/day) orally divided in 2 daily doses for 14 days

or

Co-trimoxazole, TMP, 8 mg/kg/day, with SMX, 40 mg/kg/day (maximum daily dose, 640 mg TMP and 3200 mg SMX), orally divided every 12 hours for 7 days

[1]The rationale for administering chemoprophylaxis to all household and other close contacts regardless of age and vaccination status is that immunity is not absolute and may not prevent infection. Persons with mild illness that may not be recognized as pertussis can transmit the infection.

[2]The efficacies of the alternative regimens have not been established, although other macrolides (e.g., clarithromycin) are likely to be effective.

Plague (*Yersinia pestis*)

Indication

- Persons with close exposure (within 2 meters [6.5 feet]) to persons suspected of having pneumonic plague

Recommended Regimens

Age-Group	Antibiotic
Adults ≥18 years[1]	Tetracycline, 2 g/day orally divided every (6–)12 hours for 7 days, *or* Doxycycline, 100–200 mg/day orally in two divided doses for 7 days, *or* Co-trimoxazole, TMP, 160–320 mg/day, with SMX, 1.6–3.2 g/day orally divided every 12 hours for 7 days
Children ≥9 years	Tetracycline, 25–50 mg/kg/day orally divided every (6–)12 hours for 7 days, *or* Doxycycline, 2–4 mg/kg/day orally divided every 12 hours for 7 days, *or* Co-trimoxazole, TMP, 8 mg/kg/day, with SMX, 40 mg/kg/day, orally divided every 12 hours for 7 days
Children ≥2 months	Co-trimoxazole, TMP, 8 mg/kg/day, with SMX, 40 mg/kg/day, orally divided every 12 hours for 7 days

Adapted from Centers for Disease Control and Prevention. Prevention of plague: recommendations of the Advisory Committee on Immunization Practices (ACIP). *MMWR Morb Mortal Wkly Rep* 1996:45(RR-14):12.

[1]Tetracycline or doxycycline is recommended for nonpregnant adults and children ≥8 years of age. Co-trimoxazole is recommended for pregnant women and children <8 years of age.

Rabies

Indications

- Dogs and cats
  - Healthy-appearing animals should be held for 10 days of observation, with prophylaxis (HRIG and vaccine) at the first sign of rabies in the animal; the symptomatic animal should be euthanized immediately and tested
  - Rabid or suspected rabid animals should be euthanized and tested as soon as possible; holding for observation is not recommended; vaccination is discontinued if immunofluorescent testing of the animal is negative
  - Local public health officials should be consulted for advice for unknown (escaped) dogs and cats
- Skunks, raccoons, foxes, and most other carnivores; woodchucks
  - Regard as rabid unless the geographical area is known to be free of rabies or unless the animal is proven to be negative by immunofluorescent testing; holding for observation is not recommended because of the prolonged and variable incubation of rabies in different animals, and because the clinical manifestations of rabies cannot be reliably interpreted in wild animals
- Bats
  - Bite, scratch, or mucous membrane exposure (unless the bat is available for testing and is negative for evidence of rabies)
  - Situations in the absence of a bite or scratch in which there is a reasonable probability that contact occurred (e.g., a sleeping person who awakes to find a bat in the room or an adult who witnesses a bat in the room with a previously unattended child, mentally disabled person, or intoxicated person)
- Livestock, ferrets, rodents, and lagomorphs (rabbits and hares)
  - Local public health authorities should be consulted for advice
  - Bites of squirrels, hamsters, guinea pigs, gerbils, chipmunks, rats, mice, other rodents, rabbits, and hares almost never require antirabies treatment

Recommended Regimens

Vaccination Status	Treatment	Regimen[1]
Not previously vaccinated	Local wound cleansing	Postexposure treatment begins with immediate thorough cleansing of wounds with soap and water.
	Human rabies immune globulin (HRIG; page 153)	20 IU/kg body weight. As much as possible of the **full dose** should be infiltrated into and around the wound(s), and the remainder should be administered intramuscularly at an anatomical site distant from vaccine administration. HRIG should not be administered in the same syringe as vaccine. Because HRIG may partially suppress active production of antibody, no more than the recommended dose should be given.
	Vaccine (page 86)	1.0 mL of human diploid cell vaccine rabies vaccine, adsorbed (RVA), or purified chick embryo cell culture (PCEC) vaccine administered intramuscularly (deltoid area[2]) on days 0, 3, 7, 14, and 28 (day 0 indicates the first day of treatment).
Previously vaccinated[3]	Local wound cleansing	Postexposure treatment begins with immediate thorough cleansing of all wounds with soap and water. HRIG should not be given.
	Vaccine (page 86)	1.0 mL of HDCV, RVA, or PCEC administered intramuscularly (deltoid area[2]) on days 0 and 3 (day 0 is the first day of treatment).

Adapted from Centers for Disease Control and Prevention. Human rabies—Texas and New Jersey, 1997. *MMWR Morb Mortal Wkly Rep* 1998;47:4.

[1]These regimens are applicable for all age-groups, including children.

[2]The deltoid area is the only acceptable site of vaccination for adults and older children. For younger children (<24 months of age), the anterolateral aspect of the mid-thigh may be used. Vaccine should never be administered in the gluteal area.

[3]Any person with a history of preexposure vaccination with HDCV, RVA, or PCEC; previous postexposure prophylaxis with HDCV, RVA, or PCEC; or previous vaccination with any other type of rabies vaccine and a documented history of antibody response to the prior vaccination.

Rubella

Indication

- Immune globulin: rubella antibody–negative pregnant women in the first trimester with a documented rubella exposure and who will not be terminating the pregnancy

Special Consideration

- Rubella vaccine should not be given to pregnant women

Administration

- IG, 0.55 mL/kg intramuscularly as soon as possible but within 6 days of exposure

Tetanus in Wound Management

History of Tetanus Immunization (Number of Doses)	Clean, Minor Wounds		All Other Wounds[1]	
	DTP/DTaP or Td[2]	TIG	DTP or Td	TIG
Uncertain or <3	Yes	No	Yes	Yes (page 156)
3 or more[3]	No[4]	No	No[5]	No

Adapted from Centers for Disease Control. Diphtheria, tetanus, and pertussis: recommendations for vaccine use and other preventive measures. Recommendations of the Immunization Practices Advisory Committee (ACIP). *MMWR Morb Mortal Wkly Rep* 1991;41(RR-10):21.

[1]Such as, but not limited to wounds contaminated with dirt, feces, and saliva; puncture wounds; avulsions; and wounds resulting from missiles, crushing, burns, and frostbite. TIG should be administered for tetanus-prone wounds in HIV-1–infected patients regardless of the history of tetanus immunizations.

[2]For children < 7 years of age, DTP or DTaP (if ≥3 doses of DTP/DTaP have been previously given) is preferred to tetanus toxoid alone; if pertussis vaccine is contraindicated, DT is given. For persons ≥7 years of age, Td is preferred to tetanus toxoid alone.

[3]If only 3 doses of fluid tetanus toxoid have been received, then a fourth dose of toxoid, preferably an adsorbed toxoid, should be given.

[4]Yes, if >10 years since the last dose.

[5]Yes, if >5 years since the last dose. (More frequent boosters are not needed and can accentuate adverse events.)

Tuberculosis *(Mycobacterium tuberculosis)*

SKIN TESTING[1,2]

Routine Tuberculin Skin Testing

- Annually
  - Persons infected with HIV
  - Persons in institutional settings (e.g., correctional institutions, nursing homes, and mental health facilities)
- Every 2–3 years
  - Persons with significant contact with persons at high risk of having tuberculosis (e.g., HIV-infected persons, homeless persons, residents in institutional settings [e.g., correctional institutions, nursing homes, and mental health facilities], users of illicit drugs, associates in jail or prison, migrant farm workers)
- Testing at ages 4–6 years and 11–16 years
  - Children of immigrants from regions with high prevalence of tuberculosis
  - Children with continued potential exposure
    - Continued travel to regions with high prevalence of tuberculosis
    - Continued household contact with persons from regions with high prevalence who have unknown tuberculin skin test results

Indications for Immediate Skin Testing

- Persons with radiographic or clinical findings suggesting tuberculosis
- Contacts of persons with confirmed or suspected infectious tuberculosis (contact investigation)
  - Household members diagnosed with tuberculosis

---

[1]BCG immunization is not a contraindication to tuberculin skin testing.

[2]Skin testing using the Mantoux skin test (5 tuberculin units of purified protein derivative) intradermally.

  - Household members with a recent skin test conversion from negative to positive
  - Associates in jail or prison in the last 5 years
- Persons at increased risk for progression to disease with potential exposure to tuberculosis
  - Congenital or acquired immunodeficiencies, including HIV infection
  - Diabetes mellitus
  - Chronic renal failure
  - Malnutrition
- Immigrants from regions with high prevalence of tuberculosis, especially Asia, Middle East, Africa, Latin America
- Persons with travel histories to countries with endemic tuberculosis or significant contact with persons from those countries
- Before initiation of immunosuppressive therapy

DETERMINATION OF A POSITIVE TUBERCULIN SKIN TEST[1–3]

Reaction ≥5 mm

- Close contacts of persons with known or suspected newly diagnosed infectious tuberculosis
  - Household contacts of active or previously active cases in the following situations:
    - Treatment cannot be verified as adequate before exposure
    - Treatment was initiated after contact occurred
    - Reactivation is suspected
- Persons suspected of having tuberculous disease
  - Chest radiograph consistent with active or previously active tuberculosis
  - Clinical or laboratory evidence of tuberculosis (pulmonary or extrapulmonary)
- Persons with primary or acquired immunodeficiency, including HIV infection
- Persons receiving immunosuppressive therapy (including immunosuppressive dosage of corticosteroids)

Reaction ≥10 mm

- Recent tuberculin skin test conversion (within a 2-year period) for persons <35 years of age
- Persons at increased risk of disseminated tuberculous disease
  - Age <4 years
  - Diabetes mellitus
  - Chronic renal failure
  - Malnutrition
  - Hodgkin disease or other lymphoma

---

[1]Skin testing using the Mantoux skin test (5 tuberculin units of purified protein derivative) by measuring the transverse diameter of induration (not erythema) at 48–72 hours.

[2]Regardless of previous bacille Calmette-Guérin (BCG) administration.

[3]Live-virus vaccines can interfere with an individual's response to tuberculin testing. Tuberculin skin testing, if otherwise indicated, can be done on the day that live-virus vaccines are administered or 4–6 weeks later.

- Persons with increased environmental exposure
  - Foreign-born persons and children of foreign-born persons from regions with high prevalence of tuberculosis (especially Latin America, Asia, Africa, and the Middle East)
  - Persons with significant contact with persons at high risk of having tuberculosis (e.g., HIV-infected persons, homeless persons, residents in institutional settings [e.g., correctional, nursing homes, and mental health]), users of illicit drugs, associates in jail or prison, migrant farm workers
  - Persons with travel histories to countries with endemic tuberculosis or significant contact with persons from those countries

Reaction ≥15 mm

- Recent tuberculin skin test conversion (within a 2-year period) for persons ≥35 years of age
- Children ≥4 years of age, adolescents, and adults <35 years of age[4]

---

[4]Most experts believe that the risk of drug-associated hepatitis, especially with isoniazid, may outweigh the benefits of preventive prophylaxis for adults ≥35 years of age without a history of recent exposure, recent tuberculin conversion, a chest radiograph consistent with healed tuberculosis, immunosuppression, or other risk factors.

ANTICIPATORY (PREVENTIVE) TREATMENT FOR ASYMPTOMATIC TUBERCULOUS INFECTION (POSITIVE SKIN TEST AND NO CLINICAL DISEASE)[1]

Isoniazid-Susceptible Strain Suspected or Isolated from Contact

- Children
  - Isoniazid, 10–15 mg/kg orally once daily for 9 months[2,3]

    or
  - Isoniazid, 20–30 mg/kg orally twice weekly for 9 months[2,3]
- Adults
  - Isoniazid, 300 mg orally once daily for 6–12 months[2,3]

    or
  - Isoniazid, 900 mg orally twice weekly for 6–12 months[2,3]

Isoniazid-Resistant Strain Suspected or Isolated from Contact[4]

- Children
  - Rifampin, 10–20 mg/kg orally once daily for 9 months[2]

    or
  - Rifampin, 10–20 mg/kg orally twice weekly for 9 months[2]
- Adults
  - Rifampin, 600 mg orally once daily for 6 months[2]

    with or without
  - Ethambutol, 15–25 mg/kg orally once daily for 6 months[2]

    or
  - Rifampin, 600 mg orally twice weekly for 6 months[2]

---

[1]Dosages are for patients with normal renal function.

[2]At least 6 consecutive months of therapy with good adherence should be given.

[3]Most experts recommend stopping isoniazid if the serum aminotransferase level reaches 3–5 times the upper limit of normal or patients develop symptoms of hepatitis. Isoniazid can sometimes be restarted later.

[4]These regimens are appropriate for treatment of presumed multiple-drug-resistant strains pending in vitro susceptibility studies. The regimen should be modified based on susceptibility studies of isolates from the patient or the contact. Consultation with a specialist is recommended for all patients with multiple-drug-resistant strains of *M. tuberculosis*.

Multiple-Drug-Resistant Strain Suspected or Isolated from Contact[4]

- Children
  - Pyrazinamide, 25–30 mg/kg orally once daily for 9 months
    with
  - Ethambutol, 15–25 mg/kg orally once daily for 9 months
- Adults
  - Pyrazinamide, 1.5–2.5 g orally once daily for 6 months
    with
  - Ethambutol, 15–25 mg/kg orally once daily for 6 months
    or
  - Ofloxacin, 400 mg orally twice daily for 9–12 months
    or
  - Ciprofloxacin, 750 mg orally twice daily for 9–12 months

Varicella-Zoster Virus

Indications for Immune Globulin Prophylaxis

- Candidates for postexposure prophylaxis
  - Immunocompromised children, including those who are HIV infected, without a history of chickenpox or varicella vaccination
  - Bone marrow transplant recipients, regardless of prior history of varicella or varicella vaccination in themselves or in their donors (unless varicella or zoster developed after the bone marrow transplant)
  - Susceptible pregnant women
  - Adolescents and adults known to be susceptible to chickenpox[1]
  - Hospitalized premature infants ≥28 weeks of gestation whose mothers have no history of chickenpox or who are seronegative
  - Hospitalized premature infants <28 weeks of gestation or ≤1000 g regardless of maternal history

  Who have significant exposure:
  - Household: residing in the same household
  - Playmate: face-to-face[2] indoor play
  - Hospital contact:

    Varicella: in the same 2- to 4-bed room or adjacent beds in a large ward, face-to-face[2] contact with an infectious staff member or patient, or visit by a person deemed contagious

    Zoster: intimate contact (e.g., touching or hugging) with a person deemed contagious

---

[1]Most adults with no histories or uncertain histories of chickenpox are probably immune. VZIG is not routinely recommended for healthy adults following exposure but is recommended only for adults already known to be susceptible. If varicella develops in adolescents or adults, early treatment with acyclovir is warranted.

[2]Experts differ in the duration of face-to-face contact that warrants the administration of VZIG. However, the contact should be nontransient. Some experts suggest a contact of 5 or more minutes as constituting significant exposure for this purpose; others define close contact as more than 1 hour.

- Perinatal exposure (page 210)
  - Newborn infants born to mothers with onset of chickenpox within the 5 days before delivery or within the 48 hours after delivery (page 210)

Administration

- VZIG, 125 U (one vial, approximately 1.25 mL) for each 10 kg of body weight (minimum dose 125 U; maximum dose 625 U)

Special Consideration

- Administration of live-virus vaccines is not recommended for at least 5 months following VZIG administration (page 112)

Other Infectious Agents

Empiric Therapy Following Contact or Exposure

- *Chlamydia trachomatis*
  - Mothers (and their sexual contacts) of infants with *C. trachomatis* neonatal conjunctivitis
  - Sexual contacts of persons with *C. trachomatis* infection, including nongonococcal urethritis, mucopurulent cervicitis, epididymitis, or pelvic inflammatory disease should be evaluated and treated if the last sexual contact was ≤30 days of the onset of symptoms of a symptomatic sexual contact or ≤60 days of an asymptomatic sexual contact

No Postexposure Prophylaxis Recommended Following Contact or Exposure

- Babesiosis (*Babesia* spp.)
- Cat-scratch disease (*Bartonella henselae* or *Afipia felis*)
- *Chlamydia pneumoniae*
- *Chlamydia psittaci*
  - Birds suspected to be a source of human infection should be examined by a veterinarian for evaluation, isolation (≥45 days), and management
  - All potentially contaminated housing areas should be thoroughly disinfected (70% alcohol, 1% Lysol, 1:100 dilution of household bleach) before reuse
  - Persons exposed to common sources of infection should be observed for development of fever or respiratory symptoms; persons who develop symptoms should have diagnostic tests and empiric therapy
- Hepatitis C virus (see page 169 for management protocol)
- Hepatitis D virus
- Hepatitis E virus
- Hepatitis G virus
- Human ehrlichiosis (*Ehrlichia* spp.)
- Human T cell lymphotropic virus, types I and II
- Kawasaki syndrome

- Lyme borreliosis (*Borrelia burgdorferi*)
  - The overall risk of Lyme disease in endemic areas following a tick bite is 1%–2%. Routine antimicrobial prophylaxis for Lyme borreliosis is not recommended following tick bites. Persons who develop a rash or other symptoms or signs consistent with Lyme borreliosis within 1 month following a tick bite should seek medical attention.
- *Mycoplasma pneumoniae* (respiratory tract infections)
- Rat-bite fever (*Streptococcus moniliformis* or *Spirillum minus*)
- Rocky Mountain spotted fever (*Rickettsia rickettsii)*
- *Streptococcus pneumoniae* (including antimicrobial-resistant *S. pneumoniae*)

Perinatal Prophylaxis

Ophthalmia Neonatorum (Gonococcal Conjunctivitis Caused by *Neisseria gonorrhoeae*)

Indication

- All newborns (vaginal or cesarean delivery)

Recommended Regimens[1–3]

- Silver nitrate 1% solution, 2 drops topically
  or
  Erythromycin 0.5% ophthalmic ointment, 1- to 2-cm ribbon topically
  or
  Tetracycline 1% ophthalmic ointment, 1- to 2-cm ribbon topically

Administration

- Each drug is available in single-dose ampules for use in the nursery. Administration should be within 1 hour of delivery. Before administering local prophylaxis, each eyelid should be wiped gently with sterile cotton. Two drops of a 1% silver nitrate solution are instilled into each conjunctival sac, or a 1- to 2-cm ribbon of ophthalmic antibiotic ointment is placed in each conjunctival sac and massaged gently to spread the ointment. Care should be taken to ensure that the agent reaches all parts of the conjunctival sac. The eyes should not be irrigated or flushed with saline or distilled water after

---

[1]No topical regimen has proven efficacy in preventing *Chlamydia trachomatis* neonatal conjunctivitis or extraocular disease.

[2]Silver nitrate 1% is preferred in geographical areas with penicillinase-producing *Neisseria gonorrhoeae*.

[3]An alternate regimen is penicillin G, 50,000 units intramuscularly as a single injection, but this is not recommended.

instillation of any of these agents. After 1 minute, excess solution or ointment may be wiped with sterile cotton.

Special Considerations

- Newborns whose mothers have untreated gonorrhea at the time of delivery are at high risk for infection and should receive a single dose of ceftriaxone, 125 mg, intravenously or intramuscularly (dose for low–birth weight infants: 25–50 mg/kg)
- Newborns with clinical evidence of ophthalmic or disseminated gonococcal infection should be hospitalized and treated appropriately

Group B Streptococcal Disease

Two management strategies (given in the following figures) are recommended for prevention of early-onset group B streptococcal (GBS) disease in neonates, either by prenatal screening of all women at 35–37 weeks' gestation (culture and risk factor–based approach, page 200) or by identifying newborns at risk (risk factor only–based approach, page 201).

The consensus developed by the CDC, ACOG, and AAP considers the strategy of administering chemoprophylaxis to all women with risk factors without culture screening (risk factor only–based approach) to be an equally acceptable alternative to the culture and risk factor–based approach.

PREVENTION STRATEGY FOR EARLY-ONSET GROUP B STREPTOCOCCAL DISEASE USING PRENATAL CULTURE SCREENING AT 35–37 WEEKS' GESTATION (CULTURE AND RISK FACTOR–BASED APPROACH)

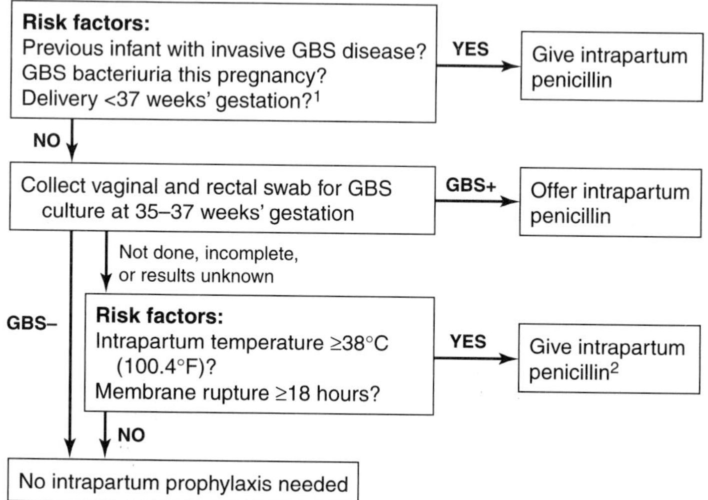

From Centers for Disease Control and Prevention. Prevention of group B streptococcal disease: A public health perspective. *MMWR Morb Mortal Wkly Rep* 1996;45(RR-7):16.

[1]No prophylaxis is needed if culture result at 35–37 weeks is known to be negative.

[2]Broad-spectrum antibiotics may be considered at the discretion of the physician based on clinical indications.

PREVENTION STRATEGY FOR EARLY-ONSET GROUP B STREPTOCOCCAL DISEASE USING RISK FACTORS WITHOUT PRENATAL SCREENING (RISK FACTOR ONLY–BASED APPROACH)

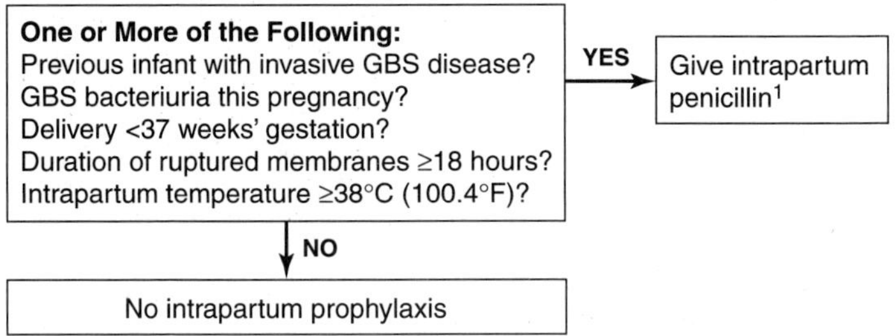

From Centers for Disease Control and Prevention. Prevention of group B streptococcal disease: a public health perspective. *MMWR Morb Mortal Wkly Rep* 1996;45(RR-7):19.

[1]Broad-spectrum antibiotics may be considered at the discretion of the physician based on clinical indications.

Consolidated Indications for Intrapartum Group B Streptococcal Prophylaxis

- Previous infant who had invasive GBS disease
- GBS bacteriuria (symptomatic or asymptomatic) during the current pregnancy
- Delivery at <37 weeks' gestation[1]
- If rectal and vaginal cultures at 35–37 weeks' gestation were done and positive for group B *Streptococcus*
- If rectal and vaginal cultures at 35–37 weeks' gestation were not done, incomplete, or unknown:
  - Intrapartum temperature ≥38.0°C (100.4°F)[2]
  - Membranes ruptured for ≥18 hours[2]

Maternal Intrapartum Antimicrobial Prophylaxis Regimens[3]

- Recommended regimen
  - Penicillin G, 5,000,000 units intravenously at onset of labor; then 2,500,000 units intravenously every 4 hours until delivery
- Alternative regimen
  - Ampicillin, 2 g intravenously at onset of labor; then 1 g intravenously every 4 hours until delivery
- For penicillin-allergic patients
  - Recommended regimen: clindamycin, 900 mg intravenously at onset of labor and every 8 hours until delivery
  - Alternative regimen: erythromycin, 500 mg intravenously at onset of labor and every 6 hours until delivery

---

Adapted from Centers for Disease Control and Prevention. Prevention of perinatal group B streptococcal disease: a public health perspective. *MMWR Morb Mortal Wkly Rep* 1996;45(RR-7):1–24.

[1]If membranes rupture at <37 weeks' gestation, and the mother has not begun labor, collect rectal and vaginal swabs for group B streptococcal culture and either (a) administer antibiotics until cultures are completed and the culture results are negative or (b) begin antibiotics only when culture results are available and are positive. No prophylaxis is needed if cultures obtained at 35–37 weeks' gestation were negative.

[2]Broader-spectrum antibiotics may be considered at the physician's discretion, based on clinical indications.

[3]If the mother is receiving treatment for amnionitis with an antimicrobial agent active against group B *Streptococcus* (e.g., ampicillin, penicillin, clindamycin, or erythromycin), additional prophylactic antibiotics are not needed.

Management of the Neonate Born to a Mother Who Received Intrapartum Antimicrobial Prophylaxis (see figure also)

- Full diagnostic laboratory evaluation (complete blood count and differential, blood culture, chest radiograph, with or without a lumbar puncture) and empiric therapy[4]
  - Signs or symptoms of sepsis in the neonate
- Limited diagnostic laboratory evaluation (complete blood count and differential, blood culture) and clinical observation for ≥48 hours[5]
  - Gestational age <35 weeks
  - Gestational age ≥35 weeks *and* duration of maternal intrapartum antimicrobial prophylaxis ≤4 hours before delivery
- No diagnostic laboratory evaluation, no therapy, and clinical observation for ≥48 hours[5]
  - Gestational age ≥35 weeks *and* duration of maternal intrapartum prophylaxis >4 hours before delivery

---

[4]The duration of therapy depends on blood culture and cerebrospinal fluid results and clinical course of the infant. If the laboratory results and clinical course are unremarkable, the duration of therapy may be as short as 48–72 hours.

[5]If sepsis is suspected clinically at any time, a full diagnostic evaluation (complete blood count and differential, blood culture, chest radiograph, with or without a lumbar puncture) and empiric therapy should be started.

SUGGESTED ALGORITHM FOR EMPIRIC MANAGEMENT OF A NEONATE BORN TO A MOTHER WHO RECEIVED INTRAPARTUM ANTIMICROBIAL PROPHYLAXIS FOR PREVENTION OF EARLY-ONSET GROUP B STREPTOCOCCAL DISEASE

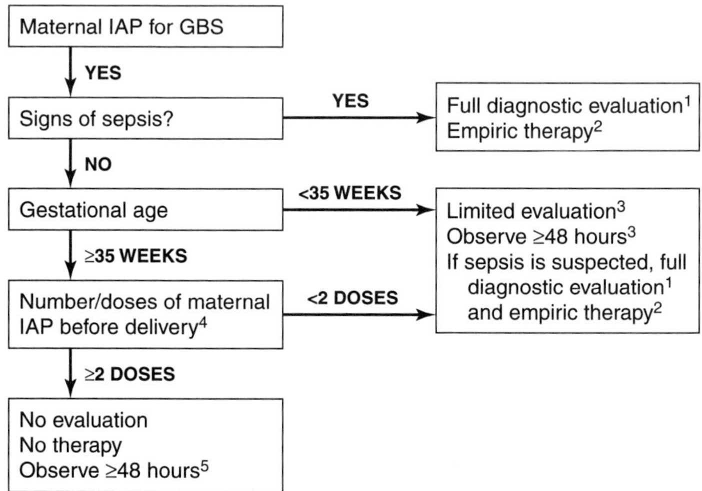

Adapted from Centers for Disease Control and Prevention. Prevention of group B streptococcal disease: a public health perspective. *MMWR Morb Mortal Wkly Rep* 1996;45(RR-7):20; Centers for Disease Control and Prevention. Erratum: vol. 45, no. RR-7. *MMWR Morb Mortal Wkly Rep* 1996;45:679.

[1]Includes CBC and differential, blood culture, and chest radiograph if respiratory symptoms are present. A lumbar puncture is performed at the discretion of the physician.

[2]Duration of therapy will vary depending on results of blood culture and CSF findings (if obtained), as well as on the clinical course of the infant. *If* laboratory results and clinical course are unremarkable, duration may be as short as 48–72 hours.

[3]CBC and differential, blood culture.

[4]Applies to penicillin or ampicillin chemoprophylaxis.

[5]Does *not* allow early discharge.

Hepatitis B

Indication: Infants born to HBsAg-positive mothers

Regimen

- HBIG, 0.5 mL intramuscularly within 12 hours of birth, *and* hepatitis B vaccine, either 5 μg of Merck vaccine (Recombivax HB) or 10 μg of SmithKline Beecham vaccine (Engerix-B), both 0.5 mL intramuscularly, within 12 hours of birth[1]
- The hepatitis B vaccine series should be completed with the same vaccine dosages at 1–2 and 6 months of age.

Follow-up: Testing for HBsAg and hepatitis B surface antibody (anti-HBs) should be at 9–15 months. If positive for anti-HBs, the child is immune to hepatitis B. If positive for HBsAg only, the parent should be counseled and the child referred to a pediatric hepatologist. If negative for both HBsAg and anti-HBs, a second complete hepatitis B vaccine series should be administered, in a 0-, 1-, and 6-month schedule followed by testing for anti-HBs 1 month after the third dose. Alternatively, testing for anti-HBs after each vaccine dose can be used to determine if subsequent doses are needed.

Special Consideration: Infants born to mothers whose HBsAg status is unknown should receive either 5 μg of Merck vaccine (Recombivax HB) or 10 μg of SmithKline Beecham vaccine (Engerix-B), both 0.5 mL intramuscularly, within 12 hours of birth. Blood should be drawn at the time of delivery to determine the mother's HBsAg status; if it is positive, the infant should receive HBIG as soon as possible (no later than 1 week after birth) and managed as for other infants born to HBsAg-positive mothers.

Adapted from Centers for Disease Control and Prevention. Protection against viral hepatitis: recommendations of the Immunization Practices Advisory Committee (ACIP). *MMWR Morb Mortal Wkly Rep* 1990;39(RR-2):15.

[1]The first dose of vaccine may be given at the same time as HBIG but at a different site. See page 59 for hepatitis B vaccine dosages and schedules.

Reduction of Perinatal HIV-1 Transmission[1]

Mothers

Antepartum: After week 14 of gestation, begin zidovudine, 100 mg orally 5 times per day

Peripartum: At the onset of labor, begin zidovudine, 2 mg/kg intravenously (loading dose) followed by continuous intravenous infusion at 1 mg/kg/hour until delivery

Infants

Postpartum: At 8–12 hours of life begin zidovudine, 2 mg/kg orally every 6 hours for 6 weeks (or zidovudine, 1.5 mg/kg intravenously every 6 hours for infants who cannot tolerate oral intake)

Adapted from Centers for Disease Control and Prevention. Public Health Service Task Force recommendations for the use of antiretroviral drugs in pregnant women infected with HIV-1 for maternal health and for reducing perinatal HIV-1 transmission in the United States. *MMWR Morb Mortal Wkly Rep* 1998;47(RR-2):2.

[1]The Pediatric AIDS Clinical Trial Group (PACTG) 076 zidovudine regimen.

CLINICAL SCENARIOS AND RECOMMENDATIONS FOR THE USE OF ANTIRETROVIRAL DRUGS[1]

Scenario 1: HIV-1–Infected Pregnant Women Who Have Not Received Prior Antiretroviral Therapy

- HIV-1–infected pregnant women must receive standard clinical, immunological, and virological evaluation. Recommendations for initiation and choice of antiretroviral therapy should be based on the same parameters used for persons who are not pregnant, although the known and unknown risks and benefits of such therapy during pregnancy must be considered and discussed.
- The three-part zidovudine (ZDV) chemoprophylaxis regimen should be recommended for all HIV-infected pregnant women to reduce the risk for perinatal transmission.
- The combination of ZDV chemoprophylaxis with additional antiretroviral drugs for treatment of HIV infection should be (1) discussed with the woman; (2) recommended for infected women whose clinical, immunological, and virological status indicates the need for treatment; and (3) offered to other infected women (although in the latter circumstance, it is not known if the combination of antenatal ZDV chemoprophylaxis with other antiretroviral drugs will provide additional benefits or risks for the infant).
- Women who are in the first trimester of pregnancy may consider delaying initiation of therapy until after 10–12 weeks' gestation.

Adapted from Centers for Disease Control and Prevention. Public Health Service Task Force recommendations for the use of antiretroviral drugs in pregnant women infected with HIV-1 for maternal health and for reducing perinatal HIV-1 transmission in the United States. *MMWR Morb Mortal Wkly Rep* 1998;47(RR-2):16–17.

[1]Discussion of treatment options and recommendations should be noncoercive, and the final decision regarding the use of antiretroviral drugs is the responsibility of the woman. A decision to decline treatment with ZDV or other drugs should not result in punitive action or denial of care. Use of ZDV should not be denied to a woman who wishes to minimize exposure of the fetus to other antiretroviral drugs and who therefore chooses to receive only ZDV during pregnancy to reduce the risk for perinatal transmission.

Scenario 2: HIV-1–Infected Women Receiving Antiretroviral Therapy during the Current Pregnancy

- HIV-1–infected women receiving antiretroviral therapy in whom pregnancy is identified after the first trimester should continue therapy.
- For women receiving antiretroviral therapy in whom pregnancy is recognized during the first trimester, the woman should be counseled regarding the benefits and potential risks of antiretroviral administration during this period, and continuation of therapy should be considered.
- If therapy is discontinued during the first trimester, all drugs should be stopped and reintroduced simultaneously to avoid the development of resistance.
- If the current therapeutic regimen does not contain ZDV, the addition of ZDV or substitution of ZDV for another nucleoside analogue antiretroviral is recommended after 14 weeks' gestation. ZDV administration is recommended for the pregnant woman during the intrapartum period and for the newborn regardless of the antepartum antiretroviral regimen.

Scenario 3: HIV-1–Infected Women in Labor Who Have Had No Prior Therapy

- Administration of intrapartum intravenous ZDV should be recommended along with the 6-week ZDV regimen for the newborn.
- In the immediate postpartum period, the woman should have appropriate assessments (e.g., CD4 cell count and HIV-1 RNA copy number) to determine whether antiretroviral therapy is recommended for her own health.

Scenario 4: Infants Born to Mothers Who Have Received No Antiretroviral Therapy during Pregnancy or Intrapartum

- The 6-week neonatal ZDV component of the ZDV chemoprophylactic regimen should be discussed with the mother and offered for the newborn.
- ZDV should be initiated as soon as possible after delivery—preferably within 12–24 hours of birth.

- Some clinicians may choose to use ZDV in combination with other antiretroviral drugs, particularly if the mother is known or suspected to have ZDV-resistant virus. However, the efficacy of this approach for prevention of transmission is unknown, and appropriate dosing regimens for neonates are incompletely defined.
- In the immediate postpartum period, the woman should undergo appropriate assessment (e.g., CD4 cell count and HIV-1 RNA copy number) to determine if antiretroviral therapy is required for her own health.

Varicella-Zoster Virus (Chickenpox)

Indication[1]

- Newborn infants born to mothers with onset of chickenpox within the 5 days before delivery or within the 48 hours after delivery

Regimen

- VZIG 125 units, 0.5 mL intramuscularly as soon as possible after birth

[1]*Perinatal* prophylaxis for varicella-zoster is indicated for infants born to mothers with primary varicella (chickenpox) in the peripartum period. *Postexposure* prophylaxis is also indicated for certain infants following exposure to varicella from any source occurring after birth, including hospitalized premature infants ≥28 weeks of gestation whose mothers have no history of chickenpox or who are seronegative, and for hospitalized premature infants <28 weeks of gestation or ≤1000 g regardless of maternal history (page 193).

Perioperative Surgical Prophylaxis

Surgical Procedure	Likely Pathogens	Recommended Antibiotic and Dose[1]
Cardiac		
Prosthetic valve, coronary artery bypass, other open heart surgery, pacemaker or defibrillator implant	Coagulase-negative staphylococci *S. aureus* *Corynebacterium* spp. Enteric gram-negative bacilli	Cefazolin, 1–2 g (pediatric dose: 12.5–25 mg/kg) intravenously,[2] *or* Cefuroxime, 1–2 g (pediatric dose: 25–50 mg/kg) intravenously,[2] *or* Vancomycin,[3] 1 g (pediatric dose: 10 mg/kg) intravenously
Gastrointestinal		
Esophageal, gastroduodenal	Enteric gram-negative bacilli Gram-positive cocci	*High risk*[4] *only:* cefazolin, 1–2 g (pediatric dose: 12.5–25 mg/kg) intravenously
Biliary tract	Enteric gram-negative bacilli *Enterococcus* spp. *Clostridium* spp.	*High risk*[5] *only:* cefazolin, 1–2 g (pediatric dose: 12.5–25 mg/kg) intravenously
Colorectal	Enteric gram-negative bacilli Anaerobes *Enterococcus* spp.	*Oral (adults):* neomycin *and* erythromycin base[6] *Parenteral* Cefoxitin 1–2 g (pediatric dose: 20–40 mg/kg) intravenously, *or* Cefotetan, 1 g (adults)
Appendectomy, nonperforated	Enteric gram-negative bacilli Anaerobes *Enterococcus* spp.	Cefoxitin, 1–2 g (pediatric dose: 20–40 mg/kg) intravenously, *or* Cefotetan, 1 g (adults) intravenously
Genitourinary	Enteric gram-negative bacilli *Enterococcus* spp.	*High risk*[7] *only:* ciprofloxacin (≥18 years of age only), 500 mg orally or 400 mg intravenously

Table continued on following page

Surgical Procedure	Likely Pathogens	Recommended Antibiotic and Dose[1]
Gynecological and Obstetrical		
Vaginal or abdominal hysterectomy	Enteric gram-negative bacilli Anaerobes Group B *Streptococcus* *Enterococcus* spp.	Cefazolin, 1–2 g (adults) intravenously, *or* Cefotetan, 1–2 g (adults) intravenously, *or* Cefoxitin, 1 g (adults) intravenously
Cesarean delivery	Same as for hysterectomy	*High risk*[8] *only*: cefazolin, 1 g (adults) intravenously after clamping umbilical cord
Abortion	Same as for hysterectomy	*First trimester, high risk*[9] *only* Aqueous penicillin G, 2 million units (adults) intravenously, *or* Doxycycline, 100 mg orally 1 hour before the abortion and 200 mg orally 1 hour after (adults) *Second trimester:* cefazolin, 1 g intravenously
Head and Neck		
Entering oral cavity or pharynx	*S. aureus* Streptococci Oral anaerobes	Cefazolin, 1–2 g (pediatric dose: 12.5–25 mg/kg) intravenously, *or* Clindamycin, 600–900 mg (pediatric dose: 10 mg/kg) intravenously *with or without* gentamicin, 1.5 mg/kg intravenously
Neurosurgery		
Craniotomy	*S. aureus* Coagulase-negative staphylococci	Cefazolin, 1–2 g (pediatric dose: 12.5–25 mg/kg) intravenously, *or* Vancomycin,[3] 1 g (pediatric dose: 10 mg/kg) intravenously

Surgical Procedure	Likely Pathogens	Recommended Antibiotic and Dose[1]
Ophthalmic	Coagulase-negative staphylococci *S. aureus* Streptococci Enteric gram-negative bacilli *Pseudomonas*	Gentamicin *or* tobramycin *or* neomycin–gramicidin–polymyxin B ophthalmic solution as multiple drops over 2–24 hours, *and* Cefazolin, 100 mg subconjunctivally at end of procedure
Orthopedic		
Total joint replacement, internal fixation of fractures	*S. aureus* Coagulase-negative staphylococci	Cefazolin, 1–2 g (pediatric dose: 12.5–25 mg/kg) intravenously, *or* Vancomycin,[3] 1 g (pediatric dose: 10 mg/kg) intravenously
Thoracic (Noncardiac)	*S. aureus* Coagulase-negative staphylococci Streptococci Enteric gram-negative bacilli	Cefazolin, 1–2 g (pediatric dose: 12.5–25 mg/kg) intravenously, *or* Cefuroxime, 1–2 g (pediatric dose: 25–50 mg/kg) intravenously, *or* Vancomycin,[3] 1 g (pediatric dose: 10 mg/kg) intravenously
Vascular		
Arterial surgery involving the abdominal aorta, a prosthesis, or a groin incision	*S. aureus* Coagulase-negative staphylococci Enteric gram-negative bacilli	Cefazolin, 1–2 g (pediatric dose: 12.5–25 mg/kg) intravenously, *or* Vancomycin,[3] 1 g (pediatric dose: 10 mg/kg) intravenously
Lower extremity amputation for ischemia	*S. aureus* Coagulase-negative staphylococci Enteric gram-negative bacilli *Clostridium* spp.	Cefazolin, 1–2 g (pediatric dose: 12.5–25 mg/kg) intravenously, *or* Vancomycin,[3] 1 g (pediatric dose: 10 mg/kg) intravenously

Table continued on following page

Surgical Procedure	Likely Pathogens	Recommended Antibiotic and Dose[1]
Contaminated Surgery[10]		
Ruptured viscus	Enteric gram-negative bacilli Anaerobes *Enterococcus* spp.	Cefoxitin, 1–2 g (pediatric dose: 20–40 mg/kg) intravenously every 6 hours, *or* Cefotetan, 1–2 g intravenously every 2 hours (adults), *with or without* Gentamicin, 1.5 mg/kg intravenously every 8 hours **Or** Clindamycin, 600 mg (pediatric dose: 10 mg/kg) intravenously every 6 hours, *and* Gentamicin, 1.5 mg/kg intravenously every 8 hours
Traumatic wound Non–bite associated	*S. aureus* Group A *Streptococcus* *Clostridium* spp.	Cefazolin, 1–2 g (pediatric dose: 12.5–25 mg/kg) intravenously divided every 8 hours[6,7]
Bite associated (dog, cat, human)	*S. aureus* Streptococci Oral anaerobes *Pasteurella multocida* (cat and dog bites) *Eikenella corrodens* (human bites)	Amoxicillin/clavulanic acid, 500 mg (pediatric dose: 10–15 mg/kg) orally every 8 hours, *or* Ampicillin/sulbactam (adults), 1–2 g (as ampicillin) intravenously every 6 hours

Adapted from *Med Lett Drugs Ther* 1997;39:98–99.

[1]Parenteral prophylactic antimicrobials should be administered as a single intravenous dose just before the operation (no more than 30 minutes preceding the initial incision). For prolonged operations, additional intraoperative doses should be administered every 4–8 hours for the duration of the procedure. Recommended doses are approximate for pediatric dosing, because standard regimens have not been established for perioperative prophylaxis in pediatrics.

[2]Some consultants recommend an additional dose when patients are removed from bypass during open-heart surgery.

[3]For hospitals in which methicillin-resistant *S. aureus* and coagulase-negative staphylococci frequently cause wound infections, or for patients allergic to penicillins or cephalosporins. Rapid intravenous administration may cause hypotension, which could be especially dangerous during induction of anesthesia. Even if the drug

is administered over 60 minutes, hypotension may occur; treatment with diphenhydramine (Benadryl and others) and further slowing of the infusion rate may be helpful. For procedures in which enteric gram-negative bacilli are possible pathogens, such as vascular surgery involving a groin incision, cefazolin should be included in the prophylaxis regimen for patients not allergic to cephalosporins.

[4]Morbid obesity, esophageal obstruction, decreased gastric acidity, or gastrointestinal motility.

[5]Age >70 years, acute cholecystitis, nonfunctioning gallbladder, obstructive jaundice, or common duct stones.

[6]After appropriate diet and catharsis, 1 g of each drug at 1 PM, 2 PM, and 11 PM the day before an 8 AM operation.

[7]Preoperative urine culture (obtained by catheterization) positive or unavailable.

[8]Active labor or premature rupture of the membranes.

[9]Patients with previous pelvic inflammatory disease, previous gonorrhea, or multiple sex partners.

[10]For contaminated or "dirty" surgery, therapy should usually be continued for about 5 days.

Infective Endocarditis Prophylaxis

Cardiac Conditions

Endocarditis Prophylaxis Recommended

- High-risk category
  - Prosthetic cardiac valves, including bioprosthetic and homograft valves
  - Previous bacterial endocarditis
  - Complex cyanotic congenital heart disease (e.g., single ventricle states, transposition of the great arteries, tetralogy of Fallot)
  - Surgically constructed systemic pulmonary shunts or conduits
- Moderate-risk category
  - Most other congenital cardiac malformations (other than as listed above and below)
  - Acquired valvar dysfunction (e.g., rheumatic heart disease)
  - Hypertrophic cardiomyopathy
  - Mitral valve prolapse with valvar regurgitation and/or thickened leaflets

Endocarditis Prophylaxis Not Recommended

- Negligible-risk category (no greater risk than the general population)
  - Isolated secundum atrial septal defect
  - Surgical repair of atrial septal defect, ventricular septal defect, or patent ductus arteriosus (without residua beyond 6 months)
  - Previous coronary artery bypass graft surgery
  - Mitral valve prolapse without valvar regurgitation
  - Physiological, functional, or innocent heart murmurs
- Previous Kawasaki disease without valvar dysfunction
- Previous rheumatic fever without valvar dysfunction
- Cardiac pacemakers (intravascular and epicardial) and implanted defibrillators

---

Adapted from Dajani AS, Taubert KA, Wilson W, et al. Prevention of bacterial endocarditis: recommendations by the American Heart Association. *JAMA* 1997; 277:1795.

Clinical Approach to Prophylaxis for Infective Endocarditis in Patients with Suspected Mitral Valve Prolapse

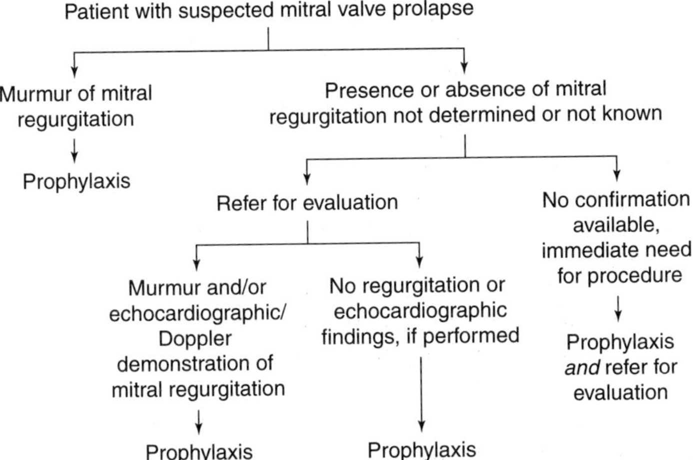

Adapted from Dajani AS, Taubert KA, Wilson W, et al: Prevention of bacterial endocarditis: recommendations by the American Heart Association. *JAMA* 1997; 277:1796.

Dental Procedures[1]

Endocarditis Prophylaxis Recommended[1]

- Dental extractions
- Periodontal procedures including surgery, scaling and root planing, probing, and recall maintenance
- Dental implant placement and reimplantation of avulsed teeth
- Endodontic (root canal) instrumentation or surgery only beyond the apex
- Subgingival placement of antibiotic fibers or strips
- Initial placement of orthodontic bands but not brackets
- Intraligamentary local anesthetic injections
- Prophylactic cleaning of teeth or implants where bleeding is anticipated

Endocarditis Prophylaxis Not Recommended[2]

- Restorative dentistry[3] (operative and prosthodontic) with or without retraction cord[2]
- Local anesthetic injections (nonintraligamentary)
- Intracanal endodontic treatment; postplacement and buildup
- Placement of rubber dams
- Postoperative suture removal
- Placement of removable prosthodontic or orthodontic appliances
- Taking of oral impressions
- Fluoride treatments
- Taking of oral radiographs
- Orthodontic appliance adjustment
- Shedding of primary teeth

Adapted from Dajani AS, Taubert KA, Wilson W, et al. Prevention of bacterial endocarditis: recommendations by the American Heart Association. *JAMA* 1997; 277:1797.

[1]Prophylaxis is recommended for patients with high- and moderate-risk cardiac conditions.

[2]Clinical judgment may indicate antibiotic use in selected circumstances that may create significant bleeding.

[3]This includes restoration of decayed teeth (filling cavities) and replacement of missing teeth.

Nondental Procedures[1]

Endocarditis Prophylaxis Recommended

- Respiratory tract
  - Tonsillectomy and/or adenoidectomy
  - Surgical operations that involve respiratory mucosa
  - Bronchoscopy with a rigid bronchoscope
- Gastrointestinal tract[1]
  - Sclerotherapy for esophageal varices
  - Esophageal stricture dilation
  - Endoscopic retrograde cholangiography with biliary obstruction
  - Biliary tract surgery
  - Surgical operations that involve intestinal mucosa
- Genitourinary tract
  - Prostatic surgery
  - Cystoscopy
  - Urethral dilation

Endocarditis Prophylaxis Not Recommended

- Respiratory tract
  - Endotracheal intubation
  - Bronchoscopy with a flexible bronchoscope, with or without biopsy[2]
  - Tympanostomy tube insertion
- Gastrointestinal tract
  - Transesophageal echocardiography[2]
  - Endoscopy with or without gastrointestinal biopsy[2]
- Genitourinary tract
  - Vaginal hysterectomy[2]
  - Vaginal delivery[2]
  - Cesarean delivery

Adapted from Dajani AS, Taubert KA, Wilson W, et al. Prevention of bacterial endocarditis: recommendations by the American Heart Association. *JAMA* 1997; 277:1797.

[1]Prophylaxis is recommended for high-risk patients; optional for medium-risk patients.

[2]Prophylaxis is optional for high-risk patients.

  - In uninfected tissue
    - Urethral catheterization
    - Uterine dilation and curettage
    - Therapeutic abortion
    - Sterilization procedures
    - Insertion or removal of intrauterine devices
- Other
  - Cardiac catheterization, including balloon angioplasty
  - Implanted cardiac pacemakers, implanted defibrillators, and coronary stents
  - Incision or biopsy of surgically scrubbed skin
  - Circumcision

Regimens for Dental, Oral, Respiratory Tract, or Esophageal Procedures

Situation	Drug	Regimen[1]
Standard general prophylaxis	Amoxicillin	Adults: 2 g Children: 50 mg/kg *Orally 1 hour before procedure*
Unable to take oral medications	Ampicillin	Adults: 2 g Children: 50 mg/kg *Intramuscularly or intravenously within 30 minutes before procedure*
Allergic to penicillin	Clindamycin	Adults: 600 mg Children: 20 mg/kg *Orally 1 hour before procedure*
	or Cephalexin[2] *or* cefadroxil[2]	Adults: 2 g Children: 50 mg/kg *Orally 1 hour before procedure*
	or Azithromycin *or* clarithromycin	Adults: 500 mg Children: 15 mg/kg *Orally 1 hour before procedure*
Allergic to penicillin and unable to take oral medications	Clindamycin	Adults: 600 mg Children: 20 mg/kg *Orally 1 hour before procedure*
	or Cefazolin[2]	Adults: 1 g Children: 25 mg/kg *Intramuscularly or intravenously within 30 minutes before procedure*

From Dajani AS, Taubert KA, Wilson W, et al. Prevention of bacterial endocarditis: recommendations by the American Heart Association. *JAMA* 1997;277:1798.

[1]Total children's dose should not exceed adult dose.

[2]Cephalosporins should not be used in individuals with immediate type of hypersensitivity reaction (urticaria, angioedema, or anaphylaxis) to penicillins.

Genitourinary and Gastrointestinal (Excluding Esophageal) Procedures

Situation	Drug	Regimen[1,2]
High-risk patients	Ampicillin plus gentamicin	*Adults:* ampicillin, 2.0 g, plus gentamicin, 1.5 mg/kg (not to exceed 120 mg), within 30 minutes of starting the procedure; 6 hours later, ampicillin, 1 g intramuscularly or intravenously, or amoxicillin, 1 g orally *Children:* ampicillin, 50 mg/kg (not to exceed 2.0 g), plus gentamicin, 1.5 mg/kg, within 30 minutes of starting the procedure; 6 hours later, ampicillin, 25 mg/kg intramuscularly or intravenously, or amoxicillin, 25 mg/kg orally
High-risk patients allergic to ampicillin/ amoxicillin	Vancomycin plus gentamicin	*Adults:* vancomycin, 1.0 g intravenously over 1–2 hours, plus gentamicin, 1.5 mg/kg intravenously or intramuscularly; complete injection/infusion within 30 minutes of starting the procedure *Children:* vancomycin, 20 mg/kg intravenously over 1–2 hours, plus gentamicin, 1.5 mg/kg intravenously or intramuscularly; complete injection/infusion within 30 minutes of starting the procedure
Moderate-risk patients	Amoxicillin *or* ampicillin	*Adults:* amoxicillin, 2.0 g orally 1 hour before procedure, or ampicillin, 2.0 g intramuscularly or intravenously within 30 minutes of starting the procedure *Children:* amoxicillin, 50 mg/kg orally 1 hour before procedure, or ampicillin, 50 mg/kg intramuscularly or intravenously within 30 minutes of starting the procedure

Situation	Drug	Regimen[1,2]
Moderate-risk patients allergic to ampicillin or amoxicillin	Vancomycin	*Adults:* vancomycin, 1.0 g intravenously over 1–2 hours; complete infusion within 30 minutes of starting the procedure *Children:* vancomycin, 20 mg/kg intravenously over 1–2 hours; complete infusion within 30 minutes of starting the procedure

From Dajani AS, Taubert KA, Wilson W, et al. Prevention of bacterial endocarditis: recommendations by the American Heart Association. *JAMA* 1997;277:1799.

[1]Total children's dose should not exceed adult dose.

[2]No second dose of vancomycin or gentamicin is recommended.

Prophylaxis for Bacterial Infections in Patients with Functional or Anatomical Asplenia

Indications

- All patients with anatomical asplenia
- Children with sickle-cell disease, beginning before 4 months of age

Duration

- For at least 2 years after splenectomy to age 6 years; prophylaxis may be continued into adulthood for high-risk patients (Immediate medical evaluation is recommended for febrile illnesses regardless of prophylaxis.)

Regimens

- Penicillin V, 125 mg orally twice daily for children <5 years of age; 250 mg orally twice daily for children ≥5 years of age and adults; *or*
- Benzathine penicillin G, 1,200,000 units intramuscularly every 3–4 weeks

Prophylaxis for Prevention of Rheumatic Fever

Primary Prevention (Treatment of Streptococcal Tonsillopharyngitis)

Indication

- All patients diagnosed with group A streptococcal tonsillopharyngitis

Recommended Regimens[1]

- Oral: penicillin V (phenoxymethyl penicillin)[2]
  - Children: 250 mg orally 2–3 times daily for 10 days
  - Adolescents and adults: 500 mg orally 3–4 times daily for 10 days *or* 500 mg orally 2 times daily for 10 days
- Parenteral: benzathine penicillin G
  - Children: 600,000 units intramuscularly once
  - Adolescents and adults: 1,200,000 units intramuscularly once
- For patients allergic to penicillin
  - Erythromycin estolate, 20–40 mg/kg/day (maximum dose, 1 g/day) orally divided 2–4 times daily for 10 days, *or*
  - Erythromycin ethylsuccinate, 40 mg/kg/day (maximum dose, 1 g/day) orally divided 2–4 times daily for 10 days

---

Adapted from Dajani A et al. Treatment of acute streptococcal pharyngitis and prevention of rheumatic fever: a statement for health professionals. Committee on Rheumatic Fever, Endocarditis, and Kawasaki Disease of the Council on Cardiovascular Disease in the Young, the American Heart Association. *Pediatrics* 1995;96:760, reproduced by permission of *Pediatrics,* vol 96, page 760, 1995; Bisno AL, Gerber MA, Gwaltney JM Jr, et al. Diagnosis and management of group A streptococcal pharyngitis: a practice guideline. *Clin Infect Dis* 1997;25:574–583.

[1]The following antibiotics are not acceptable: sulfonamides, trimethoprim, tetracyclines, and chloramphenicol.

[2]Amoxicillin is often used in place of oral penicillin V in young children. The efficacy of amoxicillin appears to be equal to that of penicillin V, and this choice is primarily based on acceptance of the taste of amoxicillin suspension.

Alternative Regimens[1]

- Oral
  - Cephalexin, 25–50 mg/kg/day (maximum dose, 2 g/day) orally divided 4 times daily for 10 days
  - Azithromycin
    - Children: 12 mg/kg/day orally once daily for 5 days
    - Adolescents and adults: 500 mg orally on day 1, then 250 mg orally on days 2–5
- Parenteral: Bicillin C-R[3](900/300), 1,200,000 units intramuscularly once

---

[3]Bicillin C-R contains 900,000 units of benzathine penicillin G and 300,000 units of procaine penicillin G.

Secondary Prevention (Prevention of Recurrent Attacks)

Indication

- All patients diagnosed with rheumatic fever require initiation of secondary prophylaxis

Regimens

- Benzathine penicillin G, 1,200,000 units intramuscularly every 3–4 weeks,[1] *or*
- Penicillin V, 250 mg orally twice daily, *or*
- Sulfadiazine, 0.5 g orally once daily for patients <60 pounds; 1.0 g orally once daily for patients >60 pounds
- For patients allergic to penicillin and sulfadiazine: erythromycin, 250 mg orally twice daily

Duration

Carditis as an Initial Manifestation of Rheumatic Fever	Duration of Secondary Prophylaxis
No carditis	5 years or until 21 years of age, whichever is longer
Carditis	10 years or well into adulthood
Carditis plus residual heart disease	10 years and at least until 40 years of age

Adapted from Dajani A et al. Treatment of acute streptococcal pharyngitis and prevention of rheumatic fever: a statement for health professionals. Committee on Rheumatic Fever, Endocarditis, and Kawasaki Disease of the Council on Cardiovascular Disease in the Young, the American Heart Association. *Pediatrics* 1995;96:762. Reproduced by permission of *Pediatrics,* vol 96, page 762, 1995.

[1]In high-risk situations, administration every 3 weeks is recommended.

Prophylaxis for *Pneumocystis carinii* Pneumonia

Children ≥4 Weeks of Age

Recommended Regimen

- Trimethoprim/sulfamethoxazole (TMP-SMX): TMP, 150 mg/m^2/day, with SMX, 750 mg/m^2/day, orally in divided doses twice daily and administered 3 times per week on consecutive days (e.g., Monday, Tuesday, and Wednesday)

Acceptable Alternative TMP-SMX Dosage Schedules

- TMP, 150 mg/m^2/day, with SMX, 750 mg/m^2/day, administered orally **as a single daily dose** 3 times per week on consecutive days (e.g., Monday, Tuesday, and Wednesday)
- TMP, 150 mg/m^2/day, with SMX, 750 mg/m^2/day, orally in divided doses twice daily and **administered 7 days per week**
- TMP, 150 mg/m^2/day, with SMX, 750 mg/m^2/day, orally in divided doses twice daily and administered 3 times per week on alternate days (e.g., Monday, Wednesday, and Friday)

Alternative Regimens if TMP-SMX is Not Tolerated[1]

- Dapsone, 2 mg/kg (not to exceed 100 mg) administered orally once daily
- Aerosolized pentamidine (children ≥5 years of age), 300 mg administered via Respirgard II nebulizer monthly

---

Adapted from Centers for Disease Control and Prevention. 1995 Revised guidelines for prophylaxis against *Pneumocystis carinii* pneumonia for children infected with or perinatally exposed to human immunodeficiency virus. *MMWR Morb Mortal Wkly Rep* 1995;44(RR-4):8.

[1]If neither dapsone nor aerosolized pentamidine is tolerated, some clinicians use intravenous pentamidine, 4 mg/kg administered every 2–4 weeks.

Adults and Adolescents

Recommended Regimen

- Trimethoprim/sulfamethoxazole (TMP-SMX), 1 double-strength tablet orally once daily

Acceptable Alternative TMP-SMX Dosage Schedules

- TMP-SMX, 1 single-strength tablet orally once daily
- TMP-SMX, 1 double-strength tablet orally three times per week

Alternative Regimens if TMP-SMX is Not Tolerated[1]

- Dapsone, 50 mg orally twice daily
- Dapsone, 100 mg orally once daily
- Dapsone, 50 mg orally once daily, *plus* pyrimethamine, 50 mg orally once weekly, *plus* leucovorin, 25 mg orally once weekly
- Dapsone, 200 mg orally once weekly, *plus* pyrimethamine, 75 mg orally once weekly, *plus* leucovorin, 25 mg orally once weekly
- Aerosolized pentamidine, 300 mg once monthly via Respirgard II nebulizer

---

[1]If neither dapsone nor aerosolized pentamidine is tolerated, some clinicians use intravenous pentamidine, 4 mg/kg administered every 2–4 weeks.

Prophylaxis for Opportunistic Disease in HIV-Infected Persons

Prophylaxis for First Episode of Opportunistic Disease in HIV-Infected Adults and Adolescents

Pathogen	Indication	Preventive Regimens	
		First Choice	Alternatives
Strongly Recommended as Standard of Care			
Pneumocystis carinii[1]	$CD4^+$ count of <200/μL *or* oropharyngeal candidiasis *or* unexplained fever for ≥2 weeks	TMP-SMX, 1 DS orally once daily, *or* TMP-SMX, 1 SS orally once daily	TMP-SMX, 1 DS orally 3 times per week; dapsone, 50 mg orally twice daily, *or* 100 mg orally once daily; dapsone, 50 mg orally once daily, *plus* pyrimethamine, 50 mg orally once weekly, *plus* leucovorin, 25 mg orally once weekly; dapsone, 200 mg orally, *plus* pyrimethamine, 75 mg orally, *plus* leucovorin, 25 mg orally once weekly; aerosolized pentamidine, 300 mg once monthly via Respirgard II nebulizer (Marquest, Englewood, Colorado)

Mycobacterium tuberculosis			
Isoniazid-sensitive[2]	Tuberculin skin test (TST) reaction ≥5 mm *or* prior positive TST result without treatment *or* contact with case of active tuberculosis	Isoniazid, 300 mg orally, *plus* pyridoxine, 50 mg orally once daily for 12 months; *or* isoniazid, 900 mg orally, *plus* pyridoxine, 50 mg orally twice weekly for 12 months	Rifampin, 600 mg orally once daily for 12 months
Isoniazid-resistant	Same; high probability of exposure to isoniazid-resistant tuberculosis	Rifampin, 600 mg orally daily for 12 months	Rifabutin, 300 mg orally daily for 12 months
Multidrug-resistant (isoniazid and rifampin)	Same; high probability of exposure to multidrug-resistant tuberculosis	Choice of drugs requires consultation with public health authorities	None
Toxoplasma gondii[3]	IgG antibody to *Toxoplasma* and $CD4^+$ count of <100/µL	TMP-SMX, 1 DS orally once daily	TMP-SMX, 1 SS orally once daily; dapsone, 50 mg orally once daily, *plus* pyrimethamine, 50 mg orally once weekly, *plus* leucovorin, 25 mg orally once weekly
Mycobacterium avium complex[4]	$CD4^+$ count of <50/µL	Clarithromycin, 500 mg orally twice daily, *or* azithromycin, 1200 mg orally once weekly	Rifabutin, 300 mg orally once daily; azithromycin, 500 mg orally once weekly, *plus* rifabutin, 300 mg orally once daily
Streptococcus pneumoniae[5]	All patients	Pneumococcal vaccine (page 83)	None
Varicella-zoster virus (VZV)	Significant exposure to chickenpox or shingles for patients who have no history of either condition or, if available, absence of antibody to VZV	Varicella-zoster immune globulin (VZIG), 5 vials (1.25 mL each) intramuscularly administered <96 hours after exposure, ideally within 48 hours (page 193)	Acyclovir, 800 mg orally 5 times per day for 3 weeks

Table continued on following page

Pathogen	Indication	Preventive Regimens: First Choice	Preventive Regimens: Alternatives
Generally Recommended			
Hepatitis B virus[6]	All susceptible (anti-HBc–negative) patients	Hepatitis B vaccine (page 56)	None
Influenza virus[6]	All patients (annually, before influenza season)	Influenza virus vaccine (page 79)	Rimantadine, 100 mg orally twice daily; *or* amantadine, 100 mg orally twice daily
Not Recommended for Most Patients (Indicated for Consideration Only in Unusual Circumstances)			
Candida species	$CD4^+$ count of <50/μL	Fluconazole, 100–200 mg orally once daily	
Bacteria	Neutropenia	Granulocyte colony-stimulating factor (G-CSF), 5–10 μg/kg subcutaneously once daily for 2–4 weeks; *or* granulocyte-macrophage colony-stimulating factor (GM-CSF), 250 μg/m^2 intravenously over 2 hours once daily for 2–4 weeks	None
Cryptococcus neoformans[7]	$CD4^+$ count of <50/μL	Fluconazole, 100–200 mg orally once daily	Itraconazole, 200 mg orally once daily
Histoplasma capsulatum[7]	$CD4^+$ count of <50/μL, endemic geographical area	Itraconazole, 200 mg orally once daily	None
Cytomegalovirus (CMV)[8]	$CD4^+$ count of <50/μL, CMV antibody positive	Oral ganciclovir, 1 g orally 3 times per day	None

Adapted from Centers for Disease Control and Prevention. 1997 USPHS/IDSA guidelines for the prevention of opportunistic infections in persons infected with human immunodeficiency virus. *MMWR Morb Mortal Wkly Rep* 1997;46(RR-12):28–29.

Anti-HBc, Antibody to hepatitis B core antigen; *CMV,* cytomegalovirus; *DS,* double-strength tablet; *SS,* single-strength tablet; *TMP-SMX,* trimethoprim-sulfamethoxazole; *TST,* tuberculin skin test.

NOTE: Information included in these guidelines may not represent Food and Drug Administration (FDA) approval or approved labeling for the particular products or indications in question. Specifically, the terms "safe" and "effective" may not be synonymous with the FDA-defined legal standards for product approval.

The Respirgard II nebulizer is manufactured by Marquest, Englewood, Colorado; Engerix-B by SmithKline Beecham, Rixensart, Belgium; and Recombivax HB by Merck & Co., West Point, Pennsylvania.

[1]Patients receiving dapsone should be tested for glucose-6-phosphate dehydrogenase deficiency. A dosage of 50 mg once daily is probably less effective than that of 100 mg once daily. The efficacy of parenteral pentamidine (e.g., 4 mg/kg/month) is uncertain. Inadequate data are available regarding the efficacy or safety of atovaquone or clindamycin-primaquine. Fansidar (sulfadoxine/pyrimethamine) is rarely used because of severe hypersensitivity reactions. TMP-SMX reduces the frequency of some bacterial infections. Patients who are being administered therapy for toxoplasmosis with sulfadiazine-pyrimethamine are protected against *Pneumocystis carinii* pneumonia and do not need TMP-SMX.

[2]Directly observed therapy is required for isoniazid (INH), 900 mg orally twice weekly; isoniazid regimens should include pyridoxine to prevent peripheral neuropathy. Rifampin should not be administered concurrently with protease inhibitors. Rifabutin, which may be administered at a reduced dose with indinavir or nelfinavir, is an option; consult an expert. Exposure to multidrug-resistant tuberculosis may require prophylaxis with two drugs; consult public health authorities. Possible regimens include pyrazinamide plus either ethambutol or a fluoroquinolone.

[3]Protection against *Toxoplasma gondii* is provided by the preferred anti–*Pneumocystis carinii* regimens. Pyrimethamine alone probably provides little, if any, protection.

[4]Rifabutin should not be administered concurrently with the protease inhibitors saquinavir or ritonavir; however, it may be administered at half the dose (150 mg orally once daily) with indinavir or nelfinavir.

[5]Vaccination should be offered to persons who have a $CD4^+$ T-lymphocyte count <200/μL, although the efficacy may be diminished. Some authorities are concerned that immunizations may stimulate the replication of HIV. However, one study showed no adverse effect of pneumococcal vaccination on patient survival.

Table continued on following page

[6]These immunizations or chemoprophylactic regimens do not target pathogens traditionally classified as opportunistic but should be considered for use in HIV-infected patients. Data are inadequate concerning clinical benefit of these vaccines in this population, although it is logical to assume that those patients who develop antibody responses will derive some protection. Some authorities are concerned that immunizations may stimulate HIV replication, although, for influenza vaccination, a large observational study of HIV-infected persons in clinical care showed no adverse effect of this vaccine, including multiple doses, on patient survival. Hepatitis B vaccine has been recommended for all children and adolescents and for all adults with risk factors for hepatitis B infection. Rimantadine and amantadine are appropriate during outbreaks of influenza A. Because of the theoretical concern that increases in HIV plasma RNA following vaccination during pregnancy might increase the risk of perinatal transmission of HIV, providers may wish to defer vaccination until after antiretroviral therapy is initiated.

[7]There may be a few unusual occupational or other circumstances under which prophylaxis should be considered; consult a specialist.

[8]Acyclovir is not protective against CMV. Valacyclovir is not recommended because of an unexplained trend toward increased mortality observed in persons who have AIDS who were being administered this drug for prevention of CMV disease.

Prophylaxis for Recurrence of Opportunistic Disease (after Chemotherapy for Acute Disease) in HIV-Infected Adults and Adolescents

		Preventive Regimens	
Pathogen	**Indication**	**First Choice**	**Alternatives**
Recommended for Life as Standard of Care			
Pneumocystis carinii	Prior *P. carinii* pneumonia	TMP-SMX, 1 DS orally once daily, *or* TMP-SMX, 1 SS orally once daily	TMP-SMX, 1 DS orally 3 times per week; dapsone, 50 mg orally twice daily, *or* 100 mg orally once daily; dapsone, 50 mg orally once daily, *plus* pyrimethamine, 50 mg orally once weekly, *plus* leucovorin, 25 mg orally once weekly; dapsone, 200 mg orally, *plus* pyrimethamine, 75 mg orally, *plus* leucovorin, 25 mg orally once weekly; aerosolized pentamidine, 300 mg once monthly via Respirgard II nebulizer (Marquest, Englewood, Colorado)
Toxoplasma gondii[1]	Prior toxoplasmic encephalitis	Sulfadiazine, 500–1000 mg orally 4 times per day, *plus* pyrimethamine, 25–75 mg orally once daily, *plus* leucovorin, 10 mg orally once daily	Clindamycin, 300–450 mg orally every 6–8 hours, *plus* pyrimethamine, 25–75 mg orally once daily, *plus* leucovorin, 10–25 mg orally 1–4 times per day

Table continued on following page

Pathogen	Indication	Preventive Regimens	
		First Choice	Alternatives
Mycobacterium avium complex[2]	Disseminated documented disease	Clarithromycin, 500 mg orally twice per day, *plus* one or more of the following: ethambutol, 15 mg/kg orally once daily; rifabutin, 300 mg orally once daily	Azithromycin, 500 mg orally once daily, *plus* one or more of the following: ethambutol, 15 mg/kg orally once daily; rifabutin, 300 mg orally once daily
Cytomegalovirus (CMV)	Prior end-organ disease	Ganciclovir, 5–6 mg/kg intravenously 5–7 days/week, *or* 1000 mg orally three times per day; *or* foscarnet, 90–120 mg intravenously once daily; *or* cidofovir, 5 mg/kg intravenously every other week; *or* (for retinitis only) ganciclovir sustained-release implant every 6–9 months	
Cryptococcus neoformans	Documented disease	Fluconazole, 200 mg orally once daily	Amphotericin B, 0.6–1 mg/kg intravenously 1–3 times per week; itraconazole, 200 mg orally once daily
Histoplasma capsulatum	Documented disease	Itraconazole, 200 mg orally twice daily	Amphotericin B, 1 mg/kg intravenously once weekly; fluconazole, 400 mg orally once daily

Coccidioides immitis	Documented disease	Fluconazole, 400 mg orally once daily	Amphotericin B, 1 mg/kg intravenously once weekly; itraconazole, 200 mg orally twice daily
Salmonella spp. (non-typhoidal)[3]	Bacteremia	Ciprofloxacin, 500 mg orally twice daily for several months	None
Recommended Only if Subsequent Episodes Are Frequent or Severe			
Herpes simplex virus	Frequent or severe recurrences	Acyclovir, 200 mg orally 3 times per day, *or* 400 mg orally twice per day	None
Candida spp. (oral, vaginal, or esophageal)	Frequent or severe recurrences	Fluconazole, 100–200 mg orally once daily	Ketoconazole, 200 mg orally once daily; itraconazole, 100 mg orally once daily

Adapted from Centers for Disease Control and Prevention. 1997 USPHS/IDSA guidelines for the prevention of opportunistic infections in persons infected with human immunodeficiency virus. *MMWR Morb Mortal Wkly Rep* 1997;46(RR-12):30–31.

DS, Double-strength tablet; *SS,* single-strength tablet; *TMP-SMX,* trimethoprim-sulfamethoxazole.

NOTE: Information included in these guidelines may not represent Food and Drug Administration (FDA) approval or approved labeling for the particular products or indications in question. Specifically, the terms "safe" and "effective" may not be synonymous with the FDA-defined legal standards for product approval.

The Respirgard II nebulizer is manufactured by Marquest, Englewood, Colorado.

[1]Pyrimethamine/sulfadiazine confers protection against *P. carinii* pneumonia as well as toxoplasmosis; clindamycin/pyrimethamine does not.

[2]Many multiple-drug regimens are poorly tolerated. Drug interactions (e.g., those seen with clarithromycin/rifabutin) can be problematic; rifabutin has been associated with uveitis, especially when administered at daily doses of >300 mg or concurrently with fluconazole or clarithromycin. Rifabutin should not be administered concurrently with the protease inhibitors saquinavir or ritonavir, but it can be administered at half dose (150 mg orally once daily) with indinavir or nelfinavir.

[3]The efficacy of eradication of *Salmonella* has been demonstrated only for ciprofloxacin.

Prophylaxis for Pneumocystis carinii *Pneumonia and CD4⁺ Monitoring for HIV-Exposed Infants and HIV-Infected Children*

Age and HIV Infection Status	PCP Prophylaxis	$CD4^+$ Monitoring
Birth to 4–6 weeks, HIV exposed	No prophylaxis	1 month
4–6 weeks to 4 months, HIV exposed	Prophylaxis (page 228)	3 months
4–12 months		
HIV infected or indeterminate	Prophylaxis (page 228)	6, 9, and 12 months
HIV infection reasonably excluded[1]	No prophylaxis	None
1–5 years, HIV infected	Prophylaxis (page 228) if $CD4^+$ count <500/μL or $CD4^+$ count <15%[2,3]	Every 3–4 months[4]
6–12 years, HIV infected	Prophylaxis (page 228) if $CD4^+$ count <200/μL or $CD4^+$ count <15%[3]	Every 3-4 months[4]

Adapted from Centers for Disease Control and Prevention. 1995 revised guidelines for prophylaxis against *Pneumocystis carinii* pneumonia for children infected with or perinatally exposed to human immunodeficiency virus. *MMWR Morb Mortal Wkly Rep* 1995;44(RR-4):6.

[1]HIV infection can be reasonably excluded among children who have had two or more negative HIV diagnostic tests (i.e., HIV culture or PCR), both of which are performed at ≥1 month of age and one of which is performed at ≥4 months of age, or two or more negative HIV IgG antibody tests performed at >6 months of age among children who have no clinical evidence of HIV disease.

[2]Children 1–2 years of age who were receiving PCP prophylaxis and had a $CD4^+$ count of <750/mL or percentage of <15% at <12 months of age should continue prophylaxis.

[3]Prophylaxis should be considered on a case-by-case basis for children who might otherwise be at risk for PCP, such as children with rapidly declining $CD4^+$ counts or percentages or children with category C conditions. Children who have had PCP should receive lifelong PCP prophylaxis.

[4]More frequent monitoring (e.g., monthly) is recommended for children whose $CD4^+$ counts or percentages are approaching the threshold at which prophylaxis is recommended.

Prophylaxis for First Episode of Opportunistic Disease in HIV-Infected Infants and Children

Pathogen	Indication	Preventive Regimens: First Choice	Preventive Regimens: Alternatives
Strongly Recommended as Standard of Care			
Pneumocystis carinii[1]	HIV-infected or HIV-indeterminate infants 1–12 months of age HIV-infected children 1–5 years of age with $CD4^+$ count <500/µL or $CD4^+$ percentage <15% HIV-infected children 6–12 years of age with $CD4^+$ count <200/µL or $CD4^+$ percentage <15%	TMP-SMX, 150/750 mg/m^2/day orally in 2 divided doses daily administered 3 times per week on consecutive days *Acceptable alternative TMP-SMX schedules (same dose):* As a single dose orally 3 times per week on consecutive days In 2 divided doses orally daily In 2 divided doses orally 3 times per week on alternate days	Aerosolized pentamidine (children ≥5 years of age), 300 mg once monthly via Respirgard II nebulizer (Marquest, Englewood, Colorado); dapsone (children ≥1 month of age), 2 mg/kg (maximum dose, 100 mg) orally once daily; pentamidine, 4 mg/kg intravenously every 2–4 weeks
Mycobacterium tuberculosis			
Isoniazid-sensitive	Tuberculin skin test (TST) reaction of ≥5 mm *or* prior positive TST result without treatment *or* contact with case of active tuberculosis	Isoniazid, 10–15 mg/kg (maximum dose, 300 mg) orally *or* intramuscularly once daily for 12 months *or* 20–30 mg/kg (maximum dose, 900 mg) orally 2 times per week for 12 months	Rifampin, 10–20 mg/kg (maximum dose, 600 mg) orally or intravenously once daily for 12 months

Table continued on following page

Pathogen	Indication	Preventive Regimens	
		First Choice	Alternatives
Isoniazid-resistant	Same; high probability of exposure to isoniazid-resistant tuberculosis	Rifampin, 10–20 mg/kg (maximum dose, 600 mg) orally or intravenously once daily for 12 months	Uncertain
Multidrug-resistant (isoniazid and rifampin)	Same; high probability of exposure to multidrug-resistant tuberculosis	Choice of drugs requires consultation with public health authorities	None
Mycobacterium avium complex	For children ≥6 years of age, $CD4^+$ count <50/µL; 2–6 years of age, $CD4^+$ count <75/µL; 1–2 years of age, $CD4^+$ count <500/µL; <1 year of age, $CD4^+$ count <750/µL	Clarithromycin, 7.5 mg/kg (maximum dose, 500 mg) orally twice per day; *or* azithromycin, 20 mg/kg (maximum dose, 1200 mg) orally once weekly	Children ≥6 years of age, rifabutin, 300 mg orally once daily; children <6 years of age, 5 mg/kg orally once daily; azithromycin, 5 mg/kg (maximum dose, 250 mg) orally once daily
Varicella-zoster virus[2]	Significant exposure to varicella with no history of varicella or zoster	Varicella-zoster immune globulin (VZIG), 125 units/10 kg (maximum dose, 625 units) intramuscularly administered ≤96 hours after exposure, ideally within 48 hours (page 193)	None
Vaccine-preventable pathogens[3]	HIV exposure/infection	Routine immunizations (page 36)	None

Generally Recommended			
Toxoplasma gondii[4]	IgG antibody to *Toxoplasma* and severe immunosuppression[5]	TMP-SMX, 150/750 mg/m^2/day orally in 2 divided doses daily	Dapsone (children ≥1 month old), 2 mg/kg, *or* 15 mg/m^2 (maximum dose, 25 mg) orally once daily, *plus* pyrimethamine, 1 mg/kg orally once daily, *plus* leucovorin, 5 mg orally every 3 days
Not Recommended for Most Patients (Indicated for Consideration Only in Unusual Circumstances)			
Invasive bacterial infections[6]	Hypogammaglobulinemia	IVIG, 400 mg/kg intravenously once monthly	None
Candida species	Severe immunosuppression[5]	Nystatin (100,000 U/mL), 4–6 mL orally every 6 hours; *or* topical clotrimazole, 10 mg orally 5 times per day	None
Cryptococcus neoformans	Severe immunosuppression[5]	Fluconazole, 3–6 mg/kg orally once daily	Itraconazole, 2–5 mg/kg orally once or twice daily
Histoplasma capsulatum	Severe immunosuppression[5] and living in an endemic geographical area	Itraconazole, 2–5 mg/kg orally once or twice daily	None
Cytomegalovirus (CMV)[7]	CMV antibody positive and severe immunosuppression[5]	Children 6–12 years old: oral ganciclovir (under investigation; consult an expert)	None

Adapted from Centers for Disease Control and Prevention. 1997 USPHS/IDSA guidelines for the prevention of opportunistic infections in persons infected with human immunodeficiency virus. *MMWR Morb Mortal Wkly Rep* 1997;46(RR-12):32–33.

Table continued on following page

CMV, cytomegalovirus; *IVIG*, intravenous immune globulin; *TMP-SMZ*, trimethoprim-sulfamethoxazole; *VZIG*, varicella-zoster immune globulin.

NOTE: Information included in these guidelines may not represent Food and Drug Administration (FDA) approval or approved labeling for the particular products or indications in question. Specifically, the terms "safe" and "effective" may not be synonymous with the FDA-defined legal standards for product approval.

The Respirgard II nebulizer is manufactured by Marquest, Englewood, Colorado.

[1]The efficacy of parenteral pentamidine (e.g., 4 mg/kg/month) is controversial. TMP-SMX, dapsone-pyrimethamine, and possibly dapsone alone appear to protect against toxoplasmosis, although data have not been prospectively collected. Daily TMP-SMX reduces the frequency of some bacterial infections. Patients receiving therapy for toxoplasmosis with sulfadiazine-pyrimethamine are protected against *Pneumocystis carinii* pneumonia (PCP) and do not need TMP-SMX.

[2]Children routinely being administered intravenous immune globulin (IVIG) should receive VZIG if the last dose of IVIG was administered >21 days before exposure.

[3]HIV-infected and HIV-exposed children should be immunized according to the childhood immunization schedule for HIV-infected children (page 36). Once an HIV-exposed child is determined not to be HIV infected, the recommended childhood immunization schedule for immunocompetent children applies (page 2).

[4]Protection against *Toxoplasma* is provided by the preferred anti–*Pneumocystis carinii* regimens. Pyrimethamine alone probably provides little, if any, protection.

[5]Severe immunosuppression is defined for HIV-infected children <13 years of age as follows:

<12 months of age $CD4^+$count <750/μL, or CD4+ percentage <15% of total lymphocytes

1–5 years of age $CD4^+$count <500/μL or CD4+ percentage <15% of total lymphocytes

6–12 years of age $CD4^+$count <200/μL or CD4+ percentage <15% of total lymphocytes

Adapted from Centers for Disease Control and Prevention. 1994 revised classification system for human immunodeficiency virus infection in children less than 13 years of age. *MMWR Morb Mortal Wkly Rep* 1994;43(RR-12).

[6]Respiratory syncytial virus (RSV) IVIG may be substituted for IVIG during the RSV season.

[7]Data on oral ganciclovir are still being evaluated; durability of effect is unclear. Acyclovir is not protective against CMV.

Prophylaxis for Recurrence of Opportunistic Disease (after Chemotherapy for Acute Disease) in HIV-Infected Infants and Children

Pathogen	Indication	Preventive Regimens	
		First Choice	**Alternatives**
Recommended for Life as Standard of Care			
Pneumocystis carinii	Prior *P. carinii* pneumonia	TMP-SMX, 150/750 mg/m^2/day orally in 2 divided doses daily administered 3 times per week on consecutive days *Acceptable alternative TMP-SMX schedules (same dose):* As a single dose orally 3 times per week on consecutive days In 2 divided doses orally daily In 2 divided doses orally 3 times per week on alternate days	Aerosolized pentamidine (children ≥5 years of age), 300 mg once monthly via Respirgard II nebulizer (Marquest, Englewood, Colorado); dapsone (children ≥1 month of age), 2 mg/kg (maximum dose, 100 mg) orally once daily; pentamidine, 4 mg/kg intravenously every 2–4 weeks
Toxoplasma gondii[1]	Prior toxoplasmic encephalitis	Sulfadiazine, 85–120 mg/kg/day orally in 2–4 divided doses, *plus* pyrimethamine, 1 mg/kg, *or* 15 mg/m^2 (maximum dose, 25 mg) orally once daily, *plus* leucovorin, 5 mg orally every 3 days	Clindamycin, 20–30 mg/kg/day orally in 4 divided doses, *plus* pyrimethamine, 1 mg/kg orally once daily, *plus* leucovorin, 5 mg orally every 3 days

Table continued on following page

Pathogen	Indication	Preventive Regimens	
		First Choice	Alternatives
Mycobacterium avium complex[2]	Prior disease	Clarithromycin, 7.5 mg/kg (maximum dose, 500 mg) orally in 2 divided doses, *plus* at least one of the following: ethambutol, 15 mg/kg (maximum dose, 900 mg) orally once daily; rifabutin, 5 mg/kg (maximum dose, 300 mg) orally once daily	
Cryptococcus neoformans	Documented disease	Fluconazole, 3–6 mg/kg orally once daily	Itraconazole, 2–5 mg/kg orally once or twice daily; amphotericin B, 0.5–1.5 mg/kg intravenously 1–3 times per week
Histoplasma capsulatum	Documented disease	Itraconazole, 2–5 mg/kg orally every 12–48 hours	Fluconazole, 3–6 mg/kg orally once daily; amphotericin B, 1.0 mg/kg intravenously once weekly
Coccidioides immitis	Documented disease	Fluconazole, 6 mg/kg orally once daily	Amphotericin B, 1.0 mg/kg intravenously once weekly
Cytomegalovirus (CMV)	Prior end-organ disease	Ganciclovir, 5 mg/kg/day intravenously daily; *or* foscarnet, 90–120 mg/kg intravenously daily; *or* (for retinitis only) ganciclovir sustained-release implant	None

Salmonella spp. (non-typhoidal)[3]	Bacteremia	TMP-SMX, 150/750 mg/m^2/day orally in 2 divided doses daily for several months	Antibiotic prophylaxis with another active agent
Recommended Only if Subsequent Episodes Are Frequent or Severe			
Invasive bacterial infections	>2 infections in a 1-year period	TMP-SMX, 150/750 mg/m^2/day orally in 2 divided doses daily; *or* IVIG, 400 mg/kg intravenously once monthly	Antibiotic prophylaxis with another active agent
Herpes simplex virus	Frequent or severe recurrences	Acyclovir, 80 mg/kg/day in 3–4 divided doses orally daily	
Candida spp.	Frequent or severe recurrences	Fluconazole, 3–6 mg/kg orally once daily; *or* ketoconazole, 5–10 mg/kg orally once or twice daily	

Adapted from Centers for Disease Control and Prevention. 1997 USPHS/IDSA guidelines for the prevention of opportunistic infections in persons infected with human immunodeficiency virus. *MMWR Morb Mortal Wkly Rep* 1997;46(RR-12):36–37.

CMV, cytomegalovirus; *IVIG,* intravenous immune globulin; *TMP-SMX,* trimethoprim-sulfamethoxazole.

NOTE: Information included in these guidelines may not represent Food and Drug Administration (FDA) approval or approved labeling for the particular products or indications in question. Specifically, the terms "safe" and "effective" may not be synonymous with the FDA-defined legal standards for product approval.

The Respirgard II nebulizer is manufactured by Marquest, Englewood, Colorado.

[1]Only pyrimethamine/sulfadiazine confers protection against *P. carinii* pneumonia as well as toxoplasmosis. Although the clindamycin plus pyrimethamine regimen is the preferred alternative for adults, it has not been tested in children. However, these drugs are safe and are used for other infections.

Table continued on following page

[2]Drug should be determined by susceptibilities of the organism isolated. Alternatives to TMP-SMX include ampicillin, chloramphenicol, or ciprofloxacin. However, ciprofloxacin is not approved for use in persons <18 years of age; therefore it should be used in children with caution and only if no alternatives exist.

[3]Antimicrobial prophylaxis should be chosen based on the microorganism and antibiotic sensitivities. TMP-SMX, if used, should be administered daily. Providers should be cautious about using antibiotics solely for this purpose because of the potential for development of drug-resistant microorganisms. IVIG may not provide additional benefit to children receiving daily TMP-SMX. Choice of antibiotic prophylaxis vs. IVIG should also involve consideration of adherence, ease of intravenous access, and cost. If IVIG is used, RSV IGIV may be substituted for IVIG during the RSV season.

Prevention of Exposure of HIV-Infected Persons to Opportunistic Pathogens

Sexual Exposures

- Patients should use a latex condom during every act of sexual intercourse to reduce the risk of acquisition of cytomegalovirus, herpes simplex virus, and human papillomavirus, as well as other sexually transmitted pathogens. Condom use also will, theoretically, reduce the risk of acquisition of human herpesvirus 8, as well as superinfection with an HIV strain that has become resistant to antiretroviral drugs, and will prevent transmission of HIV and other sexually transmitted pathogens to others. Data regarding the use and efficacy of "female condoms" are incomplete, but these devices should be considered as a risk-reduction strategy.
- Patients should avoid sexual practices that may result in oral exposure to feces (e.g., oral-anal contact) to reduce the risk of intestinal infections (e.g., cryptosporidiosis, shigellosis, campylobacteriosis, amebiasis, giardiasis, and hepatitis A and B).

Environmental and Occupational Exposures

- Certain activities or types of employment may increase the risk of exposure to tuberculosis. These include volunteer work or employment in health-care facilities, correctional institutions, and shelters for the homeless, as well as other settings identified as high risk by local health authorities. Decisions about whether to continue such activities should be made in conjunction with the health-care provider and should be based on such factors as the patient's specific duties in the workplace, the prevalence of tuberculosis in the community, and the degree to which precautions designed to prevent the transmission of tuberculosis are taken in the workplace. These decisions will affect the frequency with which the patient should be screened for tuberculosis.
- Childcare providers and parents of children in childcare are at increased risk of acquiring CMV infection, cryptosporidi-

osis, and other infections (e.g., hepatitis A, giardiasis) from children. The risk of acquiring infection can be diminished by good hygienic practices, such as hand washing after fecal contact (e.g., during diaper changing and after contact with urine or saliva). All children in childcare facilities also are at increased risk of acquiring these same infections; parents and other caretakers of HIV-infected children should be advised of this risk.

- Occupations involving contact with animals (e.g., veterinary work and employment in pet stores, farms, or slaughterhouses) may pose a risk of cryptosporidiosis, toxoplasmosis, salmonellosis, campylobacteriosis, or *Bartonella* infection. However, the available data are insufficient to justify a recommendation against work in such settings.
- Contact with young farm animals, especially animals with diarrhea, should be avoided to reduce the risk of cryptosporidiosis.
- Hand washing after gardening or other contact with soil may reduce the risk of cryptosporidiosis and toxoplasmosis.
- In areas endemic for histoplasmosis, patients should avoid activities known to be associated with increased risk, including cleaning chicken coops, disturbing soil beneath bird-roosting sites, and exploring caves.
- In areas endemic for coccidioidomycosis, when possible, patients should avoid activities associated with increased risk, including those involving extensive exposure to disturbed native soil (e.g., at excavation sites or during dust storms).

Pet-Related Exposures

- Health-care providers should advise HIV-infected persons of the potential risk posed by pet ownership. However, they should be sensitive to the possible psychological benefits of pet ownership and should not routinely advise HIV-infected persons to part with their pets. Specifically, providers should advise HIV-infected patients of the following.

General

- Veterinary care should be sought when a pet develops a diarrheal illness. If possible, HIV-infected persons should avoid contact with animals that have diarrhea. A fecal sample should be obtained from animals with diarrhea and examined for *Cryptosporidium*, *Salmonella*, and *Campylobacter*.

- When obtaining a new pet, HIV-infected patients should avoid animals <6 months of age, especially those with diarrhea. Because the hygienic and sanitary conditions in pet-breeding facilities, pet stores, and animal shelters are highly variable, the patient should be cautious when obtaining a pet from these sources. Stray animals should be avoided. Animals <6 months of age, especially those with diarrhea, should be examined by a veterinarian for *Cryptosporidium*, *Salmonella*, and *Campylobacter*.
- Patients should wash their hands after handling pets (especially before eating) and avoid contact with pets' feces to reduce the risk of cryptosporidiosis, salmonellosis, and campylobacteriosis. Hand washing for HIV-infected children should be supervised.

Cats

- Patients should consider the potential risks of cat ownership because of the risks of toxoplasmosis and *Bartonella* infection, as well as enteric infections. Those who elect to obtain a cat should adopt or purchase an animal that is >1 year of age and in good health to reduce the risk of cryptosporidiosis, *Bartonella* infection, salmonellosis, and campylobacteriosis.
- Litter boxes should be cleaned daily, preferably by an HIV-negative, nonpregnant person; if the HIV-infected patient performs this task, he or she should wash hands thoroughly afterward to reduce the risk of toxoplasmosis.
- To reduce the risk of toxoplasmosis, cats should be kept indoors, should not be allowed to hunt, and should not be fed raw or undercooked meat.
- Although declawing is not generally advised, patients should avoid activities that may result in cat scratches or bites to reduce the risk of *Bartonella* infection. Patients should also wash sites of cat scratches or bites promptly and should not allow cats to lick open cuts or wounds.
- Care of cats should include flea control to reduce the risk of *Bartonella* infection.

- Testing cats for toxoplasmosis or *Bartonella* infection is not recommended.

Birds

- Screening healthy birds for *Cryptococcus neoformans*, *Mycobacterium avium*, or *Histoplasma capsulatum* is not recommended.

Other

- Contact with reptiles (e.g., snakes, lizards, iguanas, turtles) should be avoided to reduce the risk of salmonellosis.
- Gloves should be used during the cleaning of aquariums to reduce the risk of infection with *Mycobacterium marinum*.
- Contact with exotic pets (e.g., nonhuman primates) should be avoided.

Food- and Water-Related Exposures

- Raw or undercooked eggs (including foods that may contain raw eggs [e.g., some preparations of hollandaise sauce, Caesar and certain other salad dressings, mayonnaise]); raw or undercooked poultry, meat, seafood; and unpasteurized dairy products may contain enteric pathogens. Poultry and meat should be cooked until no longer pink in the middle (internal temperature >165°F [>73.8°C]). Produce should be washed thoroughly before being eaten.
- Cross-contamination of foods should be avoided. Uncooked meats should not be allowed to come in contact with other foods. Hands, cutting boards, counters, and knives and other utensils should be washed thoroughly after contact with uncooked foods.
- Although the incidence of listeriosis is low, it is a serious disease that occurs unusually frequently among HIV-infected persons who are severely immunosuppressed. Some soft cheeses and some ready-to-eat foods (e.g., hot dogs and cold cuts from delicatessen counters) have been known to cause listeriosis. An HIV-infected person who is severely immunosuppressed and who wishes to reduce the risk of food-borne disease can prevent listeriosis by reheating these foods until they are steaming before eating them.
- Patients should not drink water directly from lakes or rivers because of the risk of cryptosporidiosis and giardiasis.

Waterborne infection may also result from swallowing water during recreational activities. Patients should avoid swimming in water that is likely to be contaminated with human or animal waste and should avoid swallowing water during swimming.

- During outbreaks or in other situations in which a community "boil water" advisory is issued, boiling water for 1 minute will eliminate the risk of acquiring cryptosporidiosis. Using submicron personal-use water filters (home/office types) and/or drinking bottled water may reduce the risk. Current data are inadequate to support a recommendation that all HIV-infected persons boil or otherwise avoid drinking tap water in nonoutbreak settings. However, persons who wish to take independent action to reduce their risk of waterborne cryptosporidiosis may choose to take precautions similar to those recommended during outbreaks. Such decisions are best made in conjunction with a health-care provider. Persons who opt for a personal-use filter or bottled water should be aware of the complexities involved in selecting the appropriate products, the lack of enforceable standards for destruction or removal of oocysts, the cost of the products, and the difficulty of using these products consistently. Patients taking precautions to avoid acquiring cryptosporidiosis from drinking water should be advised that ice made from contaminated tap water also can be a source of infection. Such persons should be aware that fountain beverages served in restaurants, bars, theaters, and other public places may also pose a risk, because these beverages, as well as the ice they may contain, are made from tap water. Nationally distributed brands of bottled or canned carbonated soft drinks are safe to drink. Commercially packaged noncarbonated soft drinks and fruit juices that do not require refrigeration until after they are opened (e.g., those that can be stored unrefrigerated on grocery shelves) also are safe. Nationally distributed brands of frozen fruit juice concentrate are safe if they are reconstituted by the user with water from a safe source. Fruit juices that must be kept refrigerated from the time they are processed to the time of consumption may be either fresh (unpasteurized) or heat treated (pasteurized);

only juices labeled as pasteurized should be considered free of risk from *Cryptosporidium.* Other pasteurized beverages and beers are also considered safe to drink. No data are available concerning survival of *Cryptosporidium* oocysts in wine.

Travel-Related Exposures

- Travel, particularly to developing countries, may carry significant risks for the exposure of HIV-infected persons to opportunistic pathogens, especially for patients who are severely immunosuppressed. Consultation with health-care providers and/or experts in travel medicine will help patients plan itineraries.
- During travel to developing countries, HIV-infected persons are at even higher risk for foodborne and waterborne infections than they are in the United States. Foods and beverages (in particular, raw fruits and vegetables, raw or undercooked seafood or meat, tap water, ice made with tap water, unpasteurized milk and dairy products, and items purchased from street vendors) may be contaminated. Items that are generally safe include steaming-hot foods, fruits that are peeled by the traveler, bottled (especially carbonated) beverages, hot coffee or tea, beer, wine, and water brought to a rolling boil for 1 minute. Treating water with iodine or chlorine may not be as effective as boiling but can be used, perhaps in conjunction with filtration, when boiling is not practical.
- Waterborne infections may result from swallowing water during recreational activities. To reduce the risk of cryptosporidiosis and giardiasis, patients should avoid swallowing water during swimming and should not swim in water that may be contaminated (e.g., with sewage or animal waste).
- Antimicrobial prophylaxis for traveler's diarrhea is not recommended routinely for HIV-infected persons traveling to developing countries. Such preventive therapy can have adverse effects and can promote the emergence of drug-resistant organisms. Nonetheless, several studies (none involving an HIV-infected population) have shown that prophylaxis can reduce the risk of diarrhea among travelers.

Under selected circumstances (e.g., those in which the risk of infection is very high and the period of travel brief), the provider and patient may weigh the potential risks and benefits and decide that antibiotic prophylaxis is warranted. For those persons to whom prophylaxis is offered, fluoroquinolones (e.g., ciprofloxacin [500 mg orally once daily]) can be considered. Trimethoprim-sulfamethoxazole (TMP-SMX) (1 double-strength tablet daily) also has been shown to be effective, but resistance to this drug is now common in tropical areas. Persons already taking TMP-SMX for prophylaxis against *Pneumocystis carinii* pneumonia (PCP) may gain some protection against travelers' diarrhea. For HIV-infected persons who are not already taking TMP-SMX, health-care providers should be cautious in prescribing this agent for prophylaxis of diarrhea because of the high rates of adverse reactions and the possible need for the agent for other purposes (e.g., PCP prophylaxis) in the future.

- All HIV-infected travelers to developing countries should carry a sufficient supply of an antimicrobial agent to be taken empirically if diarrhea develops. One appropriate regimen is ciprofloxacin, 500 mg orally twice daily for 3–7 days. Alternative antibiotics (e.g., TMP-SMX) should be considered as empirical therapy for children and pregnant women. Travelers should consult a physician if their diarrhea is severe and does not respond to empirical therapy, if their stools contain blood, if fever is accompanied by shaking chills, or if dehydration develops. Antiperistaltic agents (e.g., diphenoxylate, loperamide) are used for the treatment of diarrhea; however, they should not be used by patients with high fever or with blood in the stool, and their use should be discontinued if symptoms persist beyond 48 hours. These drugs are not recommended for children.
- Travelers should be advised about other preventive measures appropriate for anticipated exposures (e.g., chemoprophylaxis for malaria, protection against arthropod vectors, treatment with immune globulin, and vaccination). They should avoid direct contact of the skin with soil or sand (e.g., by wearing shoes and protective clothing and using towels on

beaches) in areas where fecal contamination of soil is likely.

- In general, live-virus vaccines should be avoided. An exception is measles vaccine, which is recommended for nonimmune persons. However, measles vaccine is not recommended for those who are severely immunosuppressed; immune globulin should be considered for measles-susceptible, severely immunosuppressed persons who are anticipating travel to measles-endemic countries. Inactivated (killed) poliovirus vaccine should be used instead of oral (live) poliovirus vaccine, which is contraindicated for HIV-infected persons. Persons at risk for exposure to typhoid fever should be administered an inactivated parenteral typhoid vaccine instead of the live-attenuated oral preparation. Yellow fever vaccine is a live-virus vaccine with uncertain safety and efficacy in HIV-infected persons. Travelers with asymptomatic HIV infection who cannot avoid potential exposure to yellow fever should be offered the choice of vaccination. If travel to a zone with yellow fever is necessary and vaccination is not administered, patients should be advised of the risk, instructed in methods for avoiding the bites of vector mosquitoes, and provided with a vaccination waiver letter.
- In general, killed vaccines (e.g., diphtheria-tetanus, rabies, hepatitis A, Japanese encephalitis vaccines) should be used for HIV-infected persons just as they would be used for non–HIV-infected persons anticipating travel. Preparation for travel should include a review and updating of routine vaccinations, including diphtheria-tetanus for adults and all routine immunizations for children. The currently available cholera vaccine is not recommended for persons following a usual tourist itinerary, even if travel includes countries reporting cases of cholera.
- Travelers should be informed about other area-specific risks and instructed in ways to reduce those risks. Geographically focal infections that pose a high risk to HIV-infected persons include visceral leishmaniasis (a protozoan infection transmitted by the sandfly) and several fungal infections (e.g., *Penicillium marneffei* infection, coccidioidomycosis, histo-

plasmosis). Many tropical and developing areas have high rates of tuberculosis.

Adapted from Centers for Disease Control and Prevention. 1997 USPHS/IDSA guidelines for the prevention of opportunistic infections in persons infected with human immunodeficiency virus. *MMWR Morb Mortal Wkly Rep* 1997;46(RR-12): 38–43.

Immunization and Prophylaxis for Travel

Routine Vaccinations (Should Be Up-to-date for Age)

Diphtheria, Tetanus, and Pertussis (DTP and DTaP)

- All travelers should be vaccinated with DTaP/DTP/DT/Td appropriate for age

Haemophilus influenzae *type b (Hib)*

- All travelers should be vaccinated with Hib appropriate for age

Hepatitis B

- All children through 12 years of age should be immunized routinely
- Adult international travelers who will live for more than 6 months in areas of high HBV endemicity (Southeast Asia, Africa, the Middle East, the islands of the South and Western Pacific, and the Amazon region of South America) and who will have close contact with the local population
- Adult travelers who are likely to have contact with blood from or sexual contact with residents of areas with high levels of endemic disease

Measles, Mumps, and Rubella (MMR)

- All travelers should be vaccinated with MMR appropriate for age

Poliomyelitis (eIPV and OPV)

- All travelers should be vaccinated against poliovirus appropriate for age
  - IPV for unimmunized or partially immunized adults
  - A once-per-lifetime booster (IPV or OPV) for school-age children and adults who have completed a primary series of IPV or OPV

Varicella

- All children through 12 years of age should be immunized routinely
- Adult international travelers who are known to be susceptible to varicella

Special-Use Vaccinations Indicated for Travelers

Hepatitis A

- Vaccination and/or immune globulin for hepatitis A prophylaxis is recommended for international travelers to countries with intermediate or high hepatitis A endemicity (countries other than the United States, Canada, Australia, New Zealand, Japan, Western Europe, and Scandinavia); hepatitis A vaccine may be considered for travelers ≥2 years of age to developed areas of the Caribbean
- Vaccine alone is recommended for travelers ≥2 years of age if given >14 days before travel
- If immediate protection (within 14 days) is needed, vaccine *plus* immune globulin, 0.02 mL/kg, can be administered simultaneously at separate anatomical sites
- If immune globulin is used alone for hepatitis A prophylaxis, a dose of 0.02 mL/kg by intramuscular injection into the deltoid or gluteal muscle (or the anterolateral aspect of the mid-thigh for children <24 months of age) provides short-term (1–2 months) protection; for long-term (3–5 months) protection, a dose of 0.06 mL/kg by intramuscular injection into the deltoid or gluteal muscle (or the anterolateral aspect of the mid-thigh for children <24 months of age) is administered and repeated every 5 months while continued exposure to hepatitis A virus occurs

Japanese Encephalitis

- Persons traveling for ≥1 month in endemic areas (People's Republic of China, Korea, Japan, Southeast Asia, the Indian subcontinent, and parts of Oceania) during the transmission season (May to September in temperate climates; variable in subtropical and tropical areas with rainfall, the rainy season, and the migratory patterns of avian-amplifying hosts), especially if travel will include rural areas

Meningococcus

- Patients ≥2 years of age traveling to or residing in a country with hyperendemic or epidemic meningococcal disease caused by a vaccine-preventable serogroup (A, C, Y, W-135)
- Infants ≥3 months of age traveling to an area with hyperendemic or epidemic serogroup A meningococcal disease

Rabies

- Travelers living in or visiting areas of endemic dog rabies (most countries in Central and South America, the Indian subcontinent, Southeast Asia [except Japan and Taiwan], and most of Africa) for >30 days
- Travelers to developing countries whose occupation or activities place them at frequent risk of exposure (e.g., hunters, forest rangers, taxidermists, laboratory workers, stock breeders, slaughterhouse workers, veterinarians, and spelunkers)
- If chloroquine or mefloquine is administered for malaria prophylaxis, the intramuscular vaccine should be used

Typhoid Fever

- Travelers to endemic areas of developing countries (especially Africa, Asia, and South and Central America) especially if prolonged exposure to potentially contaminated food and water is likely (The vaccine regimen should be completed at least 2 weeks [parenteral purified polysaccharide or inactivated whole-cell vaccines] or 1 week [oral live-attenuated strain of *S. typhi* Ty21a] before potential exposure.)

Yellow Fever

Yellow fever is the *only* disease for which countries may require an International Certificate of Vaccination under WHO guidelines. Some countries require a yellow fever vaccination for all travelers, whereas others only require a vaccination if a traveler is coming *from* either areas infected with yellow fever or areas where yellow fever transmission has occurred (endemic areas).

- Persons ≥9 months of age traveling to or living in areas of tropical South America and Africa where yellow fever infection is officially reported
- Persons ≥9 months of age traveling to or living in rural areas of countries that do not officially report the disease but that lie in the yellow fever endemic zone
- Infants <9 months of age and pregnant women should be considered for vaccination if traveling to areas experiencing ongoing epidemic yellow fever when travel cannot be postponed and a high level of protection against mosquito exposure is not feasible

Malaria Prophylaxis (No Vaccine Available)

- Malaria prophylaxis should be considered for travel to Mexico, Central and South America, Dominican Republic, Haiti, Africa, parts of the Middle East, Asia, and a few countries within Eastern Europe (page 266)

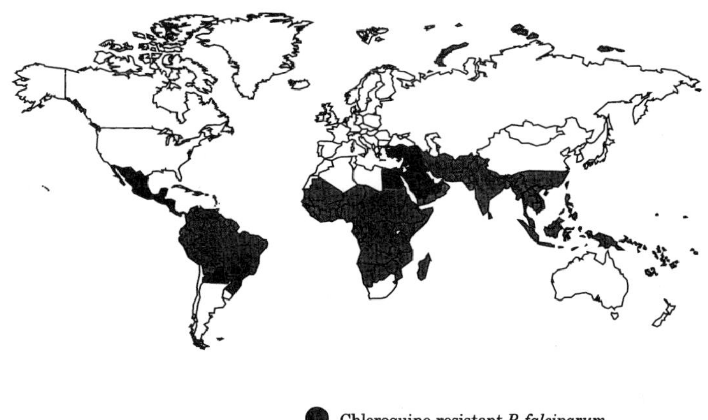

Distribution of malaria and chloroquine-resistant *Plasmodium falciparum,* 1996. From Centers for Disease Control and Prevention: *Health Information for International Travel 1996–97.* U.S. Department of Health and Human Services, Public Health Service, Atlanta, Ga, 1997.

Vaccinations Not Recommended or Required Solely for Travel (Administer if Otherwise Indicated)

Cholera

- Persons traveling to areas where local authorities require cholera vaccination
- No country requires proof of cholera vaccination as a condition for entry, and the International Certificate of Vaccination no longer provides a specific space for recording cholera vaccination

Currently no country or territory requires cholera vaccination as a condition for entry. Local authorities, however, may continue to require documentation of cholera vaccination; in such cases, a single dose of vaccine is sufficient to satisfy local requirements. Persons following the usual tourist itinerary who use standard accommodations in countries reporting cholera are at virtually no risk of infection.

- Cholera vaccine induces incomplete, unreliable protection of short duration, and its use therefore is not recommended; cholera vaccine is only approximately 50% effective in reducing clinical illness, with the greatest protection during the first 2 months following immunization, and does not protect against non-O1 serotypes of cholera, such as *V. cholerae* O139
- Travelers to cholera-infected areas should take appropriate food precautions (page 270)
- Vaccination against cholera cannot prevent the introduction of the infection into a country; the World Health Assembly therefore amended the International Health Regulations in 1973 so that cholera vaccination is no longer required of any traveler

Bacille-Calmette-Guérin (BCG)

Influenza

Plague

Pneumococcus

Tickborne Encephalitis

- Vaccines may be obtained in Europe, but available data do not support recommendation for use in travelers; travelers should be advised to avoid tick-infested areas and to protect themselves from tick bites by limiting exposure, dressing appropriately, and using insect repellents (page 269)

Vaccinia (Smallpox)

- The global eradication of smallpox was declared by WHO in 1980; smallpox vaccination is no longer indicated and may be dangerous to those who are vaccinated and those in close contact with vaccinees

Summary of Immunization and Prophylaxis for Travel[1]

Vaccine	North America, Northern or Southern Europe, Scandinavia, Australia, New Zealand, Japan	Eastern Mediter-ranean, North Africa	Tropical Africa	Middle East	Asia, Including India	Mexico, Central and South America	Caribbean and Pacific islands
Routine Vaccinations							
DTP/DT							
Children	DTP/DT up-to-date for all travel						
Adults	Td booster up-to-date for all travel						
H. influenzae type b							
Children	Up-to-date for all travel						
Adults	Not necessary unless otherwise recommended (page 52)						
Hepatitis B							
Children	Up-to-date for all travel (universal immunization recommended through age 12 years)						
Adults		Yes, for prolonged visit (>6 months)				Yes	Yes, for prolonged visit (>6 months)

Table continued on following page

Vaccine	North America, Northern or Southern Europe, Scandinavia, Australia, New Zealand, Japan	Eastern Mediter-ranean, North Africa	Tropical Africa	Middle East	Asia, Including India	Mexico, Central and South America	Caribbean and Pacific islands
MMR							
Children	Up-to-date for all travel (as early as 6 months if necessary [will need 2 additional doses if first dose given <12 months of age], with 2 doses for all children >12 months of age [page 60])						
Adults	Not necessary unless otherwise recommended (page 60)						
Polio							
Children	Up-to-date for all travel						
Adults	A once-per-lifetime booster (OPV or IPV) for all travel						
Varicella							
Children	Up-to-date for all travel (universal immunization recommended through age 12 years)						
Adults	Yes, if known to be seronegative						
Vaccinations for Travel							
Hepatitis A		Yes					Optional
Typhoid fever		Yes					
Yellow fever[2]			Central, West, East Africa			Equatorial countries	

Rabies			Yes, for prolonged visit (>30 days; >2 weeks for spelunkers)				Yes, for prolonged visit (>30 days; >2 weeks for spelunkers)
Meningococcus		North Africa	Yes, for prolonged visit or during outbreaks; recommended during winter months	Recommended during outbreaks; required for pilgrimage to Mecca	Parts of India and Nepal, particularly if trekking	Recommended during outbreaks	
Japanese encephalitis					Yes, for prolonged visit		
Cholera	Not recommended for any travel						

[1]No vaccine is required for travel to the United States.

[2]Yellow fever is the *only* disease for which countries may require an International Certificate of Vaccination under WHO guidelines. Some countries require a yellow fever vaccination for all travelers, whereas others only require a vaccination if a traveler is coming *from* either areas infected with yellow fever or areas where yellow fever transmission has occurred (endemic areas).

Chemoprophylaxis of Malaria

Regimen[1,2] (and Timing)	Pediatric Dosage	Adult Dosage
Prophylaxis for Travel to Areas Where Chloroquine-Resistant Malaria Has Not Been Reported		
Recommended regimen		
Chloroquine phosphate (1–2 weeks before exposure and continuing weekly while in malarious area and for 4 weeks after last exposure)	5 mg/kg base (8.3 mg/kg salt) up to adult dose orally once per week[3]	300 mg base (500 mg salt) orally once per week
Alternative regimen		
Hydroxychloroquine sulfate (1–2 weeks before exposure and continuing weekly while in malarious area and for 4 weeks after last exposure)	5 mg/kg base (6.5 mg/kg salt) up to adult dose orally once per week	310 mg base (400 mg salt) orally once per week
Prophylaxis for Travel to Areas with Chloroquine-Resistant Malaria		
Recommended regimen[4]		
Mefloquine (1–2 weeks before exposure and continuing weekly while in malarious area and for 4 weeks after last exposure)	<15 kg: 4.6 mg/kg base (5 mg/kg salt) orally once per week 15–19 kg: ¼ tablet orally once per week 20–30 kg: ½ tablet orally once per week 31–45 kg: ¾ tablet orally once per week >45 kg: 1 tablet orally once per week	228 mg base (250 mg salt, U.S. formulation) orally once per week *or* 250 mg base (other countries) orally once per week
Alternative regimens[4]		
Doxycycline (1–2 days before exposure and continuing daily while in malarious area and for 4 weeks after last exposure) *or*	>8 years: 2 mg/kg up to adult dose orally once per day	100 mg orally once per day

Regimen[1,2] (and Timing)	Pediatric Dosage	Adult Dosage
Chloroquine phosphate[3]	Same as above for chloroquine phosphate	Same as above for chloroquine phosphate
plus in Africa south of the Sahara		
Proguanil[5] (not licensed in the United States; available in Canada, Europe, and Africa) (1–2 days before exposure and continuing daily while in malarious area and for 4 weeks after last exposure, in combination with weekly chloroquine)	<2 years: 50 mg orally once per day 2–6 years: 100 mg orally once per day 7–10 years: 150 mg orally once per day >10 years: 200 mg orally once per day	200 mg orally once per day
plus presumptive self-treatment (all areas)		
Pyrimethamine-sulfadoxine (Fansidar) (Single dose for self-treatment of febrile illness when using chloroquine ± proguanil when medical care is not immediately available[6])	2–12 months (5–10 kg): ½ tablet orally in 1 dose 1–3 years (11–20 kg): 1 tablet orally in 1 dose 4–8 years (21–30 kg): 1½ tablets orally in 1 dose 9–14 years (31–45 kg): 2 tablets orally in 1 dose >14 years (>45 kg): 3 tablets orally in 1 dose	3 tablets (total of 75 mg pyrimethamine and 1500 mg sulfadoxine) orally in 1 dose

Table continued on following page

Regimen[1,2] (and Timing)	Pediatric Dosage	Adult Dosage
Individuals with Prolonged Exposure *(e.g., Missionaries, Peace Corps Volunteers) from Areas Endemic for* **Plasmodium** vivax *and* P. ovale *(Almost All Areas Except Haiti) or with Intense* P. vivax *Exposure (e.g., Papua New Guinea)*		
Primaquine[7] (Daily during the last 2 weeks of chemoprophylaxis for prevention of "relapsing" malaria ["terminal prophylaxis"])	0.3 mg/kg base (0.5 mg/kg salt) up to adult dose orally once per day for 14 days	15-mg base (26.3-mg salt) orally once per day for 14 days

[1]Review drug contraindications and side effects before use. No drug regimen guarantees protection against malaria. Travelers to countries with a risk of malaria should be advised to avoid mosquito bites by using personal protective measures (page 269).

[2]Malaria in a pregnant woman increases the risk of maternal death, miscarriage, stillbirth, and low birth weight with associated risk of neonatal death. Travel during pregnancy to a malarious area, especially areas of chloroquine-resistant malaria, should be discouraged. Chloroquine prophylaxis can be taken in areas where chloroquine-resistant malaria has not been reported. In areas with chloroquine-resistant malaria, chloroquine and proguanil prophylaxis should be taken during the first 3 months of pregnancy; mefloquine prophylaxis may be taken from the fourth month of pregnancy. Doxycycline and primaquine should not be used in pregnancy. Pregnant women should seek medical help if malaria is suspected. Quinine is the drug of choice for presumptive self-treatment if medical care is not immediately available; medical help must still be sought as soon as possible. Pyrimethamine-sulfadoxine should not be used in pregnant women at term or in infants younger than 2 months. Nonpregnant women of childbearing potential should avoid pregnancy during the period of mefloquine or doxycycline prophylaxis and for 3 months after mefloquine prophylaxis is stopped and 1 week after doxycycline prophylaxis is stopped.

[3]A better-tasting chloroquine syrup is available in some European countries.

[4]The CDC recommends mefloquine for persons at risk of infection who are traveling to the Indian subcontinent, the Philippines, and part of Indonesia, whereas the WHO recommends chloroquine plus proguanil or no prophylaxis.

[5]Failures in prophylaxis with chloroquine and proguanil have been reported in travelers to sub-Saharan Africa.

[6]Continue the chloroquine ± proguanil with presumptive interim self-treatment. Presumptive self-treatment is not necessary for most travelers taking mefloquine or doxycycline. Resistance to pyrimethamine-sulfadoxine (Fansidar) may limit the effectiveness in some areas. Presumptive self-treatment should not delay seeking medical attention and should not be used when medical care is readily available. Seek medical help immediately for a child who develops a febrile illness; the symptoms of malaria in children may not be typical. In infants, malaria should be suspected even in nonfebrile illness.

[7]Glucose-6-phosphate dehydrogenase (G6PD) level should be checked before prescribing primaquine.

Protection from Infections While Traveling

Protection from Tick- and Mosquito-Borne Infections

- Avoid tick- and mosquito-infested areas
  - Avoid outdoor activities during dusk and dawn
  - Avoid excrement of wild animals
  - Avoid grassy or marshy woodland areas during summer and fall
  - Remain in air-conditioned or well-screened areas, especially at night and while sleeping
  - Use aerosol indoor spray insecticides at sundown
- Dress appropriately
  - Wear long-sleeved shirts and long trousers that cover the arms and legs, with trousers tucked into shoes or boots
  - Do not wear sandals
- Use insect repellents
  - Apply *N,N*-diethyl-*m*-toluamide (DEET) to clothing and exposed skin (do not apply to cuts, wounds, irritated skin, eyes, mouth, or underclothing)
  - Apply permethrin to clothing
  - Wash after returning indoors
- Remove ticks
  - Regularly inspect for ticks, especially after outdoor activities
  - Remove ticks by grasping the tick close to the skin, as close as possible to the mouth parts, using blunt tweezers to steadily pull the tick outward
  - Avoid squeezing, twisting, or crushing the tick, especially the tick's bloated abdomen
  - The application of heat or suffocation methods (e.g., petrolatum jelly, nail polish) is of no benefit and may cause the tick to regurgitate into the bloodstream
  - Prophylactic antibiotics are not indicated

Protection from Other Infections

- Avoid sexual contact

Travelers' Diarrhea

Beverage and Food Precautions

Recommended beverages and foods

- Breast milk
- Boiled water
- Canned or bottled carbonated beverages, beer, and wine with the outside of the container wiped clean and dry
- Drink mixes, tea, coffee, or powdered formula made with boiled water
- Personally peeled or freshly cooked fruits or vegetables
- Freshly prepared hot foods and cereals
- Breads and dry baked goods
- Hot noodles, rice, or pasta
- Well-cooked meat or fish, eaten while hot

Generally safe beverages and foods

- Meals prepared in private family homes
- Food that has been cooked and that is still hot
- Fruits peeled yourself
- Jams, jellies, or honey
- Preserved, dried, salted, or pickled foods
- Tap water that is uncomfortably hot to touch
- Water purified by vigorous boiling (for a few minutes at high altitudes) or chemical disinfectant tablets with either iodine (preferred) or chlorine. For disinfection with iodine use tincture of iodine or tetraglycine hydroperiodide (e.g., Globaine, Potable-Aqua). If the water is cloudy, then strain it through a clean cloth, and double the amount of disinfectant used. Adding a pinch of salt or pouring the water from one container to another will improve the taste. The CDC makes no recommendations for portable filters because of lack of independently verified results of efficacy

Beverages and foods to avoid

- Cloudy or tap water (Do not brush teeth with tap water.)
- Unpasteurized or unirradiated milk or dairy products
- Ice or ice products, such as flavored ice desserts
- Raw fruits or vegetables
- Salads

- Undercooked or raw meat, fish, or shellfish
- Fish or shellfish in regions with known outbreaks of biotoxins (e.g., ciguatoxin)
  - Tropical reef fish (red snapper, amberjack, grouper, and sea bass) if caught on tropical reefs rather than the open ocean
  - Barracuda and puffer fish are often toxic and should be avoided
  - Highest risk areas include the islands of the West Indies and the tropical Pacific and Indian Oceans
- Reheated foods
- Food from street vendors

Antimicrobial Prophylaxis and Treatment

Prophylactic antibiotics

- Not routinely recommended
- Bismuth subsalicylate (Pepto-Bismol): 2 oz or 2 tablets orally 4 times daily may be effective for prevention but is not recommended for periods of more than 3 weeks or in children, adolescents, or pregnant women[1]

Presumptive self-treatment

- Initiated at first symptoms of diarrhea, nausea, bloating, or urgency
- Adults (≥18 years of age)
  - Ciprofloxacin (500 mg), norfloxacin (400 mg), or ofloxacin (300 mg) orally twice daily for 3 days
  - Co-trimoxazole (160 mg TMP–800 mg SMX) orally twice daily for 3 days
- Children (≥2 months of age)
  - Co-trimoxazole (4 mg TMP–20 mg SMX/kg/dose, maximum 160 mg TMP–800 mg SMX) orally twice daily for 3 days

---

[1]There is concern about taking such large amounts of bismuth and salicylate. This should not be used by persons with intolerance to salicylates, renal insufficiency, or gout; those taking anticoagulants, probenecid, or methotrexate; or those who take salicylates for other reasons.

Symptomatic treatment

- Replacement of fluids and salts lost in diarrheal stools
- WHO oral rehydration solution (ORS) packets are available at stores or pharmacies in almost all developing countries
- Prompt medical evaluation is indicated for disease persisting >3 days, bloody stools, fever >102°F or chills, persistent vomiting, or moderate to severe dehydration, especially in a young child or pregnant woman
- Loperamide (Imodium) reduces diarrhea by 80%; bismuth salicylate (Pepto-Bismol) reduces diarrhea by 50%. Not for diarrhea with blood or mucus or with high fever. Limit use to 2 days.

Drug and Age	Dosage
Loperamide	
≥12 years	4 mg, then 2 mg after each unformed stool, not to exceed 8 mg/day
9–11 years	2 mg, then 1 mg after each unformed stool, not to exceed 6 mg/day
6–8 years	1 mg, then 1 mg after each unformed stool, not to exceed 4 mg/day
<6 years	Not recommended
Bismuth salicylate[1]	
≥12 years	30 mL or 2 tablets as often as every 30 minutes for 8 doses, with no more than 8 doses in 24 hours
9–11 years	15 mL or 1 tablet, as above
6–8 years	10 mL or ⅔ of a tablet, as above
3–5 years	5 mL or ⅓ of a tablet, as above
<3 years	Not recommended

[1]There is concern about taking such large amounts of bismuth and salicylate. This should not be used by persons with intolerance to salicylates, renal insufficiency, or gout; those taking anticoagulants, probenecid, or methotrexate; or those who take salicylates for other reasons.

Isolation Precautions in Hospitals

Types of Precautions

Category	Hand Washing for Patient Contact	Single Room	Masks	Gowns and Gloves
Standard Precautions[1]	Yes	No	No	No
Transmission-Based Precautions				
Airborne	Yes	Yes, with negative-pressure ventilation	Yes	No
Droplet	Yes	Yes[2]	Yes, for close contact (<3 feet)	No
Contact	Yes	Yes[2]	No	Yes

[1]Standard Precautions are indicated for all patients and apply to (1) blood; (2) all body fluids, secretions, and excretions except sweat; (3) nonintact skin; and (4) mucous membranes.

[2]A single room is preferred but not required for crib-confined patients. Cohorting of children infected with the same pathogen is acceptable.

Type and Duration of Precautions for Certain Infections and Conditions

Infection/Condition	Precautions: Type[1]	Precautions: Duration[2]
Abscess		
Draining, major[3]	C	DI
Draining, minor or limited[4]	S	
Acquired immunodeficiency syndrome[5]	S	
Actinomycosis	S	
Adenovirus infection in infants and young children	D, C	DI
Amebiasis	S	
Anthrax		
Cutaneous	S	
Pulmonary	S	
Antibiotic-associated colitis (see *Clostridium difficile*)		
Arthropod-borne viral encephalitides (eastern, western, Venezuelan equine encephalomyelitis; St. Louis, California encephalitis)	S[6]	

Table continued on following page

Infection/Condition	Precautions	
	Type[1]	Duration[2]
Arthropod-borne viral fevers (dengue, yellow fever, Colorado tick fever)	S[6]	
Ascariasis	S	
Aspergillosis	S	
Babesiosis	S	
Blastomycosis, North American (cutaneous or pulmonary)	S	
Botulism	S	
Bronchiolitis (see Respiratory infectious disease in infants and young children)		
Brucellosis (undulant, Malta, Mediterranean fever)	S	
Campylobacter gastroenteritis (see Gastroenteritis)		
Candidiasis, all forms including mucocutaneous	S	
Cat-scratch fever (benign inoculation lymphoreticulosis)	S	
Cellulitis, uncontrolled drainage	C	DI
Chancroid (soft chancre)	S	
Chickenpox (varicella; see F[7] for varicella exposure)	A, C	F[7]
Chlamydia trachomatis		
Conjunctivitis	S	
Genital	S	
Respiratory	S	
Cholera (see Gastroenteritis)		
Closed-cavity infection		
Draining, limited or minor	S	
Not draining	S	
Clostridium		
C. botulinum	S	
C. difficile	C	DI
C. perfringens		
Food poisoning	S	
Gas gangrene	S	
Coccidioidomycosis (valley fever)		
Draining lesions	S	
Pneumonia	S	
Colorado tick fever	S	
Congenital rubella	C	F[8]
Conjunctivitis		
Acute bacterial	S	
Chlamydia	S	
Gonococcal	S	
Acute viral (acute hemorrhagic)	C	DI
Coxsackievirus disease (see Enteroviral infections)		
Creutzfeldt-Jakob disease	S[9]	

Infection/Condition	Precautions Type[1]	Duration[2]
Croup (see Respiratory infectious disease in infants and young children)		
Cryptococcosis	S	
Cryptosporidiosis (see Gastroenteritis)		
Cysticercosis	S	
Cytomegalovirus infection, neonatal or immunosuppressed	S	
Decubitus ulcer, infected		
Major[3]	C	DI
Minor or limited[4]	S	
Dengue	S[6]	
Diarrhea, acute—infective etiology suspected (see Gastroenteritis)		
Diphtheria		
Cutaneous	C	CN[10]
Pharyngeal	D	CN[10]
Ebola viral hemorrhagic fever	C[11]	DI
Echinococcosis (hydatidosis)	S	
Echovirus (see Enteroviral infections)		
Encephalitis or encephalomyelitis (see specific etiological agents)		
Endometritis	S	
Enterobiasis (pinworm disease, oxyuriasis)	S	
Enterococcus species (see Multidrug-resistant organisms if epidemiologically significant or vancomycin resistant)		
Enterocolitis, *Clostridium difficile*	C	DI
Enteroviral infections		
Adults	S	
Infants and young children	C	DI
Epiglottitis caused by *Haemophilus influenzae*	D	U[24 hr]
Epstein-Barr virus infection, including infectious mononucleosis	S	
Erythema infectiosum (see also Parvovirus B19)	S	
Escherichia coli gastroenteritis (see Gastroenteritis)		
Food poisoning		
Botulism	S	
Clostridium perfringens or *welchii*	S	
Staphylococcal	S	
Furunculosis—staphylococcal		
Infants and young children	C	DI
Gangrene (gas gangrene)	S	

Table continued on following page

Infection/Condition	Precautions	
	Type[1]	Duration[2]
Gastroenteritis		
Campylobacter species	S[12]	
Cholera	S[12]	
Clostridium difficile	C	DI
Cryptosporidium species	S[12]	
Escherichia coli		
Enterohemorrhagic O157:H7	S[12]	
Diapered or incontinent	C	DI
Other species	S[12]	
Giardia lamblia	S[12]	
Rotavirus	S[12]	
Diapered or incontinent	C	DI
Salmonella species (including *S. typhi*)	S[12]	
Shigella species	S[12]	
Diapered or incontinent	C	DI
Vibrio parahaemolyticus	S[12]	
Viral (if not covered elsewhere)	S[12]	
Yersinia enterocolitica	S[12]	
German measles (rubella)	D	F[13]
Giardiasis (see Gastroenteritis)		
Gonococcal ophthalmia neonatorum (gonorrheal ophthalmia, acute conjunctivitis of newborn)	S	
Gonorrhea	S	
Granuloma inguinale (donovanosis, granuloma venereum)	S	
Guillain-Barré syndrome	S	
Hand, foot, and mouth disease (see Enteroviral infections)		
Hantavirus pulmonary syndrome	S	
Helicobacter pylori	S	
Hemorrhagic fevers (e.g., Lassa, Ebola)	C[11]	DI
Hepatitis, viral		
Hepatitis A	S	
Diapered or incontinent patients	C	F[14]
Hepatitis B—HBsAg positive	S	
Hepatitis C and other unspecified non-A, non-B	S	
Hepatitis E	S	
Herpangina (see Enteroviral infections)		
Herpes simplex *(Herpesvirus hominis)*		
Encephalitis	S	
Neonatal[15] (see F[15] for perinatal exposure)	C	DI
Mucocutaneous, disseminated or primary, severe	C	DI
Mucocutaneous, recurrent (skin, oral, genital)	S	

Infection/Condition	Precautions	
	Type[1]	Duration[2]
Herpes zoster (varicella-zoster)		
Localized in immunocompromised patient, or disseminated	A, C	DI[16]
Localized in normal patient	S[16]	
Histoplasmosis	S	
Hookworm disease (ancylostomiasis, uncinariasis)	S	
Human immunodeficiency virus (HIV) infection[5]	S	
Impetigo	C	U[24 hr]
Infectious mononucleosis	S	
Influenza	D[17]	DI
Kawasaki syndrome	S	
Lassa fever	C[11]	DI
Legionnaire disease	S	
Leprosy	S	
Leptospirosis	S	
Lice (pediculosis)	C	U[24 hr]
Listeriosis	S	
Lyme disease	S	
Lymphocytic choriomeningitis	S	
Lymphogranuloma venereum	S	
Malaria	S[6]	
Marburg virus disease	C[11]	DI
Measles (rubeola), all presentations	A	DI
Melioidosis, all forms	S	
Meningitis	S	
Aseptic (nonbacterial or viral meningitis [see Enteroviral infections])		
Bacterial, gram-negative enteric, in neonates	S	
Fungal	S	
Haemophilus influenzae, known or suspected	D	U[24 hr]
Listeria monocytogenes	S	
Neisseria meningitidis (meningococcal), known or suspected	D	U[24 hr]
Pneumococcal	S	
Tuberculosis[18]	S	
Other diagnosed bacterial	S	
Meningococcal pneumonia	D	U[24 hr]
Meningococcemia (meningococcal sepsis)	D	U[24 hr]
Molluscum contagiosum	S	
Mucormycosis	S	
Multidrug-resistant organisms, infection or colonization[19]		
Gastrointestinal	C	CN

Table continued on following page

Infection/Condition	Precautions Type[1]	Duration[2]
Multidrug-resistant organisms, infection or colonization[19] *Continued*		
Respiratory	C	CN
Pneumococcal	S	
Skin, wound, or burn	C	CN
Mumps (infectious parotitis)	D	F[20]
Mycobacteria, nontuberculosis (atypical)		
Pulmonary	S	
Wound	S	
Mycoplasma pneumonia	D	DI
Necrotizing enterocolitis	S	
Nocardiosis, draining lesions or other presentations	S	
Norwalk agent gastroenteritis (see Gastroenteritis, viral)		
Orf	S	
Parainfluenza virus infection, respiratory in infants and young children	C	DI
Parvovirus B19	D	F[21]
Pediculosis (lice)	C	U[24 hr]
Pertussis (whooping cough)	D	F[22]
Pinworm infection	S	
Plague		
Bubonic	S	
Pneumonic	D	U[72 hr]
Pleurodynia (see Enteroviral infections)		
Pneumonia		
Adenovirus	D, C	DI
Bacterial not listed elsewhere (including gram-negative bacterial)	S	
Burkholderia cepacia in cystic fibrosis (CF) patients, including respiratory tract colonization	S[23]	
Chlamydia	S	
Fungal	S	
Haemophilus influenzae		
Adults	S	
Infants and children (any age)	D	U[24 hr]
Legionella	S	
Meningococcal	D	U[24 hr]
Multidrug-resistant bacterial (see Multidrug-resistant organisms)	S	
Mycoplasma (primary atypical pneumonia)	D	DI
Pneumococcal	S	
Multidrug-resistant (see Multidrug-resistant organisms)		

Infection/Condition	Precautions	
	Type[1]	Duration[2]
Pneumonia *Continued*		
Pneumocystis carinii	S[24]	
Pseudomonas cepacia (see *Burkholderia cepacia*)	S[23]	
Staphylococcus aureus	S	
Streptococcus, group A		
Adults	S	
Infants and young children	D	U[24 hr]
Viral		
Adults	S	
Infants and young children[5]	C	DI
Poliomyelitis	S	
Psittacosis (ornithosis)	S	
Q fever	S	
Rabies	S	
Rat-bite fever (*Streptobacillus moniliformis* disease, *Spirillum minus* disease)	S	
Relapsing fever	S	
Resistant bacterial infection or colonization (see Multidrug-resistant organisms)		
Respiratory infectious disease, acute (if not covered elsewhere)		
Adults	S	
Infants and young children[5]	C	DI
Respiratory syncytial virus infection in infants, young children, and immunocompromised adults	C	DI
Reye syndrome	S	
Rheumatic fever	S	
Rickettsial fevers, tickborne (Rocky Mountain spotted fever, tickborne typhus fever)	S	
Rickettsialpox (vesicular rickettsiosis)	S	
Ringworm (dermatophytosis, dermatomycosis, tinea)	S	
Ritter disease (staphylococcal scalded skin syndrome)	S	
Rocky Mountain spotted fever	S	
Roseola infantum (exanthema subitum)	S	
Rotavirus infection (see Gastroenteritis)		
Rubella (German measles; see also Congenital rubella)	D	F[13]
Salmonellosis (see Gastroenteritis)		
Scabies	C	U[24 hr]
Scalded skin syndrome, staphylococcal (Ritter disease)	S	
Schistosomiasis (bilharziasis)	S	
Shigellosis (see Gastroenteritis)		
Sporotrichosis	S	

Table continued on following page

Infection/Condition	Precautions	
	Type[1]	Duration[2]
Spirillum minus disease (rat-bite fever)	S	
Staphylococcal disease *(S. aureus)*		
Skin, wound, or burn		
Major[3]	C	DI
Minor or limited[4]	S	
Enterocolitis	S[12]	
Multidrug-resistant (see Multidrug-resistant organisms)		
Pneumonia	S	
Scalded skin syndrome	S	
Toxic shock syndrome	S	
Streptobacillus moniliformis disease (rat-bite fever)	S	
Streptococcal disease (group A streptococcus)		
Skin, wound, or burn		
Major[3]	C	U[24 hr]
Minor or limited[4]	S	
Endometritis (puerperal sepsis)	S	
Pharyngitis in infants and young children	D	U[24 hr]
Pneumonia in infants and young children	D	U[24 hr]
Scarlet fever in infants and young children	D	U[24 hr]
Streptococcal disease (group B streptococcus), neonatal	S	
Streptococcal disease (not group A or B) unless covered elsewhere	S	
Multidrug-resistant (see Multidrug-resistant organisms)		
Strongyloidiasis	S	
Syphilis		
Skin and mucous membrane, including congenital, primary, secondary	S	
Latent (tertiary) and seropositivity without lesions	S	
Tapeworm disease		
Hymenolepis nana	S	
Taenia solium (pork)	S	
Other	S	
Tetanus	S	
Tinea (fungus infection, dermatophytosis, dermatomycosis, ringworm)	S	
Toxoplasmosis	S	
Toxic shock syndrome (staphylococcal disease)	S	
Trachoma, acute	S	
Trench mouth (Vincent angina)	S	
Trichinosis	S	

Infection/Condition	Precautions	
	Type[1]	Duration[2]
Trichomoniasis	S	
Trichuriasis (whipworm disease)	S	
Tuberculosis		
Extrapulmonary, draining lesion (including scrofula)	S	
Extrapulmonary, meningitis[18]	S	
Pulmonary (confirmed or suspected) or laryngeal disease	A	F[25]
Skin test positive with no evidence of current pulmonary disease	S	
Tularemia		
Draining lesion	S	
Pulmonary	S	
Typhoid *(Salmonella typhi)* fever (see Gastroenteritis)		
Typhus, endemic and epidemic	S	
Urinary tract infection (including pyelonephritis), with or without urinary catheter	S	
Varicella (chickenpox)	A, C	F[7]
Vibrio parahaemolyticus (see Gastroenteritis)		
Vincent angina (trench mouth)	S	
Viral diseases		
Respiratory (if not covered elsewhere)		
Adults	S	
Infants and young children[5]	C	DI
Whooping cough (pertussis)	D	F[22]
Wound infections		
Major[3]	C	DI
Minor or limited[4]	S	
Yersinia enterocolitica gastroenteritis (see Gastroenteritis)		
Zygomycosis (phycomycosis, mucormycosis)	S	
Zoster (varicella-zoster)		
Localized in immunocompromised patient, disseminated	A, C	DI[16]
Localized in normal patient	S[16]	

Adapted from Garner JS, the Hospital Infection Control Practices Advisory Committee. Guideline for isolation precautions in hospitals. *Infect Control Hosp Epidemiol* 1996;17:73–80.

[1] *A*, Airborne; *C*, contact; *D*, droplet; *S*, standard; when *A*, *C*, and *D* are specified, also use *S*.

Table continued on following page

[2]*CN,* Until off antibiotics and culture negative; *DH,* duration of hospitalization; *DI,* duration of illness (with wound lesions, *DI* means until they stop draining); *U,* until time specified in hours (hr) after initiation of effective therapy; *F,* see footnote number.

[3]No dressing or dressing does not contain drainage adequately.

[4]Dressing covers and contains drainage adequately.

[5]Pulmonary tuberculosis should be suspected in an HIV-infected patient or a patient at high risk for HIV infection presenting with cough, fever, and pulmonary infiltrate in any lung location.

[6]Install screens in windows and doors in endemic areas.

[7]Maintain precautions until all lesions are crusted. The average incubation for varicella is 10 to 16 days, with a range of 10 to 21 days. After exposure, use varicella-zoster immune globulin (VZIG) when appropriate, and discharge susceptible patients if possible. Place exposed susceptible patients on Airborne Precautions beginning 10 days after exposure and continuing until 21 days after last exposure (up to 28 days if VZIG has been given). Susceptible persons should not enter the room of patients on precautions if other immune caregivers are available.

[8]Place infant on precautions during any admission until 1 year of age, unless nasopharyngeal and urine cultures are negative for virus after 3 months of age.

[9]Additional special precautions are necessary for handling and decontamination of blood, body fluids and tissues, and contaminated items from patients with confirmed or suspected disease. See latest College of American Pathologists (Northfield, Illinois) guidelines (www.cap.org/html/publications/cjd.html) or other references.

[10]Until two cultures taken at least 24 hours apart are negative.

[11]Call state health department and CDC for specific advice about management of a suspected case. See Centers for Disease Control and Prevention. Update: management of patients with suspected viral hemorrhagic fever—United States. *MMWR Morb Mortal Wkly Rep* 1995;44:475–479.

[12]Use Contact Precautions for diapered or incontinent children <6 years of age for duration of illness.

[13]Until 7 days after onset of rash.

[14]Maintain precautions in infants and children <3 years of age for duration of hospitalization; in children 3 to 14 years of age, until 2 weeks after onset of symptoms; and in others, until 1 week after onset of symptoms.

[15]For infants delivered vaginally or by cesarean and if mother has active infection and membranes have been ruptured for more than 4 to 6 hours.

[16]Persons susceptible to varicella are also at risk for developing varicella when exposed to patients with herpes zoster lesions; therefore susceptible persons should not enter the room if other immune caregivers are available.

[17]The "Guideline for Prevention of Nosocomial Pneumonia" (see Selected Bibliography, page 299) recommends surveillance, vaccination, antiviral agents, and use of private rooms with negative air pressure as much as feasible for patients for whom influenza is suspected or diagnosed. Many hospitals encounter logistical difficulties and physical plant limitations when admitting multiple patients with suspected influenza during community outbreaks. If sufficient private rooms are unavailable, consider cohorting patients or, at the very least, avoid room sharing

with high-risk patients. See "Guideline for Prevention of Nosocomial Pneumonia" (see Selected Bibliography, page 299) for additional prevention and control strategies.

[18]Patients should be examined for evidence of current (active) pulmonary tuberculosis. If evidence exists, additional precautions are necessary (see Tuberculosis).

[19]Resistant bacteria judged by the infection control program, based on current state, regional, or national recommendations, to be of special clinical and epidemiological significance.

[20]For 9 days after onset of swelling.

[21]Maintain precautions for duration of hospitalization when chronic disease occurs in an immunodeficient patient. For patients with transient aplastic crisis or red-cell crisis, maintain precautions for 7 days.

[22]Maintain precautions until 5 days after patient is placed on effective therapy.

[23]Avoid cohorting or placement in the same room with a cystic fibrosis patient who is not infected or colonized with *B. cepacia.* Persons with cystic fibrosis who visit or provide care and are not infected or colonized with *B. cepacia* may elect to wear a mask when within 3 feet of a colonized or infected patient.

[24]Avoid placement in the same room with an immunocompromised patient.

[25]Discontinue precautions *only* when the patient is on effective therapy, is improving clinically, and has three consecutive negative sputum smears collected on different days, or tuberculosis is ruled out. Also see CDC "Guidelines for Preventing the Transmission of Tuberculosis in Health-Care Facilities" (see Selected Bibliography, page 299).

Selected Bibliography

Vaccinations

Routine Childhood Immunization Schedule

Ad hoc Working Group for the Development of Standards for Pediatric Immunization Practices. Standards for pediatric immunization practices. *JAMA* 1993;269:1817–1822.

American Academy of Family Physicians. Summary of policy recommendations for periodic health examination. Kansas City, Mo: American Academy of Family Physicians, November 1996. (AAFP order no. 962, reprint no. 510.)

American Academy of Pediatrics, Committee on Infectious Diseases. Peter G, ed. *1997 Red book: report of the Committee on Infectious Diseases*. 24th ed. Elk Grove Village, Ill: American Academy of Pediatrics, 1997.

American Academy of Pediatrics, Committee on Infectious Diseases. Recommended childhood immunization schedule—United States, January-December 1998. *Pediatrics* 1998;101:154–157.

American Academy of Pediatrics, Committee on Practice and Ambulatory Medicine. Implementation of the immunization policy (S94–26). *Pediatrics* 1995;96:360–361.

American Academy of Pediatrics, Committee on Practice and Ambulatory Medicine. Recommendations for preventive pediatric health care. *Pediatrics* 1995;96:373–374.

Centers for Disease Control and Prevention. General recommendations on immunization: recommendations of the Advisory Committee on Immunization Practices (ACIP). *MMWR Morb Mortal Wkly Rep* 1994;43(RR-1):1–38.

Centers for Disease Control and Prevention. Update: vaccine side effects, adverse reactions, contraindications, and precautions. Recommendations of the Advisory Committee on Immunization Practices (ACIP). *MMWR Morb Mortal Wkly Rep* 1996;45(RR-12):1–35. (Published erratum appears in Centers for Disease Control and Prevention. Erratum: vol. 45, no. RR-12. *MMWR Morb Mortal Wkly Rep* 1997; 46:227.)

Centers for Disease Control and Prevention. Recommended childhood immunization schedule—United States, 1998. *MMWR Morb Mortal Wkly Rep* 1998;47:8–12.

Gershon AA, Gardner P, Peter G, Nichols K, Orenstein W: Quality standards for immunization: guidelines from the Infectious Diseases Society of America. *Clin Infect Dis* 1997;25:782–786.

Immunization Schedule for Children Behind in Immunization

Centers for Disease Control and Prevention. General recommendations on immunization: recommendations of the Advisory Committee on Immunization Practices (ACIP). *MMWR Morb Mortal Wkly Rep* 1994;43(RR-1).

Routine Immunizations

Diphtheria, Tetanus, and Pertussis (DTP/DTaP/DT/Td)

American Academy of Pediatrics, Committee on Infectious Diseases. The relationship between pertussis vaccine and central nervous system sequelae: continuing assessment. *Pediatrics* 1996;97:279–281.

American Academy of Pediatrics, Committee on Infectious Diseases. Acellular pertussis vaccine: recommendations for use as the initial series in infants and children. *Pediatrics* 1997;99:282–288.

Centers for Disease Control and Prevention. Diphtheria, tetanus, and pertussis: recommendations for vaccine use and other preventive measures: recommendations of the Immunizations Practices Advisory Committee (ACIP). *MMWR Morb Mortal Wkly Rep* 1991;40(RR-10): 1–28.

Centers for Disease Control and Prevention. Pertussis vaccination: use of acellular pertussis vaccines among infants and young children. Recommendations of the Immunization Practices Advisory Committee (ACIP). *MMWR Morb Mortal Wkly Rep* 1997;46(RR-7):1–25. (Published erratum appears in Centers for Disease Control and Prevention. Erratum: vol. 46, no. RR-7. *MMWR Morb Mortal Wkly Rep* 1997; 46:706.)

Haemophilus influenzae type b (Hib)

American Academy of Pediatrics, Committee on Infectious Diseases. *Haemophilus influenzae* type b vaccines: recommendations for immunization with recently and previously licensed vaccines. *Pediatrics* 1993;92:480–488.

Centers for Disease Control. *Haemophilus* b conjugate vaccines for prevention of *Haemophilus influenzae* type b disease among infants and children two months of age and older: recommendations of the Immunization Practices Advisory Committee (ACIP). *MMWR Morb Mortal Wkly Rep* 1991;40(RR-1):1–7.

Centers for Disease Control and Prevention. Recommendations for use of *Haemophilus* b conjugate vaccines and a combined diphtheria, tetanus, pertussis, and *Haemophilus* b vaccine. *MMWR Morb Mortal Wkly Rep* 1993;42(RR-13):1–15.

Hepatitis B

American Academy of Pediatrics, Committee on Infectious Diseases. Universal hepatitis B immunization. *Pediatrics* 1992;89:795–800. (Published erratum appears in *Pediatrics* 1992;90:715).

American Academy of Pediatrics, Committee on Infectious Diseases. Update on timing of hepatitis B vaccination for premature infants and for children with lapsed immunization. *Pediatrics* 1994;94:403–404.

Centers for Disease Control and Prevention. Hepatitis B virus: a comprehensive strategy for eliminating transmission in the United States through universal childhood vaccination: recommendations of the Immunization Practices Advisory Committee (ACIP). *MMWR Morb Mortal Wkly Rep* 1991;40(RR-13):1–25.

Centers for Disease Control and Prevention. Update: recommendations to prevent hepatitis B virus transmission—United States. *MMWR Morb Mortal Wkly Rep* 1995;44:574–575.

Measles, Mumps, and Rubella (MMR)

American Academy of Pediatrics, Committee on Infectious Diseases. Revised recommendations on rubella vaccine. *Pediatrics* 1980;65: 1182–1184.

American Academy of Pediatrics, Committee on Infectious Diseases. Personal and family history of seizures and measles immunization. *Pediatrics* 1987;80:741–742.

American Academy of Pediatrics, Committee on Infectious Diseases. Measles: reassessment of the current immunization policy. *Pediatrics* 1990;84:1110–1113. (Published erratum appears in *Pediatrics* 1990; 85:714.)

American Academy of Pediatrics, Committee on Infectious Diseases. Recommended timing of routine measles immunization for children who have recently received immune globulin preparations. *Pediatrics* 1994;93:682–685.

American Academy of Pediatrics, Committee on Infectious Diseases. Age of routine administration of the second dose of measles-mumps-rubella vaccine. *Pediatrics* 1998;101:129–133.

Centers for Disease Control and Prevention. Measles, mumps, and rubella vaccine use and strategies for measles, rubella, and congenital rubella syndrome elimination and mumps control: recommendations of the Immunization Practices Advisory Committee (ACIP). *MMWR Morb Mortal Wkly Rep* 1998;47(RR-8):1–57.

Poliomyelitis

American Academy of Pediatrics, Committee on Infectious Diseases. Poliomyelitis prevention: recommendations for use of inactivated poliovirus vaccine and live oral poliovirus vaccine. *Pediatrics* 1997; 99:300–305.

Centers for Disease Control and Prevention. Poliomyelitis prevention in the United States: introduction of a sequential vaccination schedule of inactivated poliovirus vaccine followed by oral poliovirus vaccine. Recommendations of the Advisory Committee on Immunization Practices (ACIP). *MMWR Morb Mortal Wkly Rep* 1997;46(RR-3):1–25.

Varicella-zoster Virus

American Academy of Pediatrics, Committee on Infectious Diseases. Recommendations for the use of live attenuated varicella vaccine. *Pediatrics* 1995;95:791–796. (Published erratum appears in *Pediatrics* 1995;96[1, pt. 1]:preceding 151 and following 171.)

Centers for Disease Control and Prevention. Prevention of varicella: recommendations of the Advisory Committee on Immunization Practices (ACIP). *MMWR Morb Mortal Wkly Rep* 1996;45(RR-11):1–36.

Combination Vaccines

Comvax

Centers for Disease Control. FDA approval for infants of a *Haemophilus influenzae* type b conjugate and hepatitis B (recombinant) combined vaccine. *MMWR Morb Mortal Wkly Rep* 1997;46:107–109.

Tetramune

Centers for Disease Control and Prevention. Recommendations for use of *Haemophilus* b conjugate vaccines and a combined diphtheria, tetanus, pertussis, and *Haemophilus* b vaccine. *MMWR Morb Mortal Wkly Rep* 1993;42(RR-13):1–15.

TriHIBit

Centers for Disease Control and Prevention. Recommendations for use of *Haemophilus* b conjugate vaccines and a combined diphtheria, tetanus, pertussis, and *Haemophilus* b vaccine. *MMWR Morb Mortal Wkly Rep* 1993;42(RR-13):1–15.

Frequently Used Special Vaccines

Hepatitis A

American Academy of Pediatrics, Committee on Infectious Diseases. Prevention of hepatitis A infections: guidelines for use of hepatitis A vaccine and immune globulin. *Pediatrics* 1996;98:1207–1215.

Centers for Disease Control and Prevention. Prevention of hepatitis A through active or passive immunization: recommendations of the Advisory Committee on Immunization Practices (ACIP). *MMWR Morb Mortal Wkly Rep* 1996;45(RR-15):1–30. (Published erratum appears in Centers for Disease Control and Prevention. Erratum: vol. 45, no. RR-15. *MMWR Morb Mortal Wkly Rep* 1997;46:588.)

Influenza

Each year influenza vaccine recommendations are reviewed and amended to reflect updated information concerning influenza activity in the United States for the preceding influenza season and to provide information on the vaccine available for the upcoming influenza season. These recommendations are published annually in *MMWR Morb Mortal Wkly Rep*, usually during May or June. See www.pedid.uthscsa.edu for updated information.

Centers for Disease Control and Prevention. Prevention and control of influenza: recommendations of the Advisory Committee on Immunization Practices (ACIP). *MMWR Morb Mortal Wkly Rep* 1998;47(RR-6):1–26.

Centers for Disease Control and Prevention. Update: influenza activity—United States and worldwide. 1997–98 season, and composition of the 1998–99 influenza vaccine. *MMWR Morb Mortal Wkly Rep* 1998; 47:280–284.

Meningococcus

Centers for Disease Control and Prevention. Control and prevention of meningococcal disease: recommendations of the Advisory Committee on Immunization Practices (ACIP). *MMWR Morb Mortal Wkly Rep* 1997;46(RR-5):1–10.

Centers for Disease Control and Prevention. Control and prevention of serogroup C meningococcal disease: evaluation and management of suspected outbreaks: recommendations of the Advisory Committee on Immunization Practices (ACIP). *MMWR Morb Mortal Wkly Rep* 1997;46(RR-5):13–21.

Pneumococcus

American Academy of Pediatrics, Committee on Infectious Diseases. Recommendations for using pneumococcal vaccine in children. *Pediatrics* 1985;75:1153–1158.

Centers for Disease Control and Prevention. Prevention of pneumococcal disease: recommendations of the Advisory Committee on Immunization Practices. *MMWR Morb Mortal Wkly Rep* 1997;46 (RR-8):1–24.

Rabies

Centers for Disease Control and Prevention. Rabies prevention—United States, 1991: recommendations of the Immunization Practices Advisory Committee (ACIP). *MMWR Morb Mortal Wkly Rep* 1991;40 (RR-3):1–19.

Centers for Disease Control and Prevention. Availability of new rabies vaccine for human use. *MMWR Morb Mortal Wkly Rep* 1998;47:12, 19.

Centers for Disease Control and Prevention. Compendium of animal rabies control, 1998: National Association of State Public Health Veterinarians, Inc. *MMWR Morb Mortal Wkly Rep* 1998;47:(RR-9):1–9.

Typhoid Fever (*Salmonella typhi*)

Centers for Disease Control and Prevention. Typhoid immunization: recommendations of the Advisory Committee on Immunization Practices (ACIP). *MMWR Morb Mortal Wkly Rep* 1994;34(RR-14):1–7.

Infrequently Used Special Vaccines

Bacille-Calmette-Guérin (BCG)

Centers for Disease Control and Prevention. The role of BCG vaccine in the prevention and control of tuberculosis in the United States: a joint statement by the Advisory Council for the Elimination of Tuberculosis and the Advisory Committee on Immunization Practices. *MMWR Morb Mortal Wkly Rep* 1996;45(RR-4):1–18.

Cholera

Centers for Disease Control. Cholera vaccine: recommendations of the Advisory Committee on Immunization Practices (ACIP). *MMWR Morb Mortal Wkly Rep* 1988;37:617–624.

Japanese Encephalitis

Centers for Disease Control. Inactivated Japanese encephalitis virus vaccine: recommendations of the Advisory Committee on Immunization Practices (ACIP). *MMWR Morb Mortal Wkly Rep* 1993;42 (RR-1):1–15.

Plague

Centers for Disease Control and Prevention: Prevention of plague: recommendations of the Advisory Committee on Immunization Practices (ACIP). *MMWR Morb Mortal Wkly Rep* 1996;45(RR-14):1–15.

Vaccinia (Smallpox)

Centers for Disease Control. Vaccinia (smallpox) vaccine: recommendations of the Advisory Committee on Immunization Practices (ACIP). *MMWR Morb Mortal Wkly Rep* 1991;40(RR-14):1–10.

Yellow Fever

Centers for Disease Control. Yellow fever vaccine: recommendations of the Advisory Committee on Immunization Practices (ACIP). *MMWR Morb Mortal Wkly Rep* 1990:39(RR-6):1–6.

Immunization of Adolescents

American Academy of Pediatrics, Committee on Infectious Diseases. Immunization of adolescents: recommendations of the Advisory Committee on Immunization Practices, the American Academy of Pediatrics, the American Academy of Family Physicians, and the American Medical Association. *Pediatrics* 1997;99:479–488.

American Medical Association. Rationale and recommendations: infectious diseases. In Elster AB, Kuznets NJ, eds. *AMA guidelines for adolescent preventive services (GAPS): recommendations and rationale.* Chicago: Williams & Wilkins, 1994:165–171.

Centers for Disease Control and Prevention. Immunization of adolescents: recommendations of the Advisory Committee on Immunization Practices, the American Academy of Pediatrics, the American Academy of Family Physicians, and the American Medical Association. *MMWR Morb Mortal Wkly Rep* 1996;45(RR-13):1–16.

Immunization of Adults

American College of Physicians Task Force on Adult Immunization and Infectious Diseases Society of America. *Guide for adult immunization.* 3rd ed. Philadelphia: American College of Physicians, 1994.

Centers for Disease Control. Update on adult immunization: recommendations of the Immunization Practices Advisory Committee (ACIP). *MMWR Morb Mortal Wkly Rep* 1991;40(RR-12):1–94.

Fedson DS, for the National Vaccine Advisory Committee. Adult immunization: summary of the National Vaccine Advisory Committee report. *JAMA* 1994;272:1133–1137.

Gershon AA, Gardner P, Peter G, Nichols K, Orenstein W. Quality standards for immunization: guidelines from the Infectious Diseases Society of America. *Clin Infect Dis* 1997;25:782–786.

Immunization of Health-Care Workers

Centers for Disease Control and Prevention. Immunization of health-care workers: recommendations of the Advisory Committee on Immunization Practices (ACIP) and the Hospital Infection Control Practices Advisory Committee (HICPAC). *MMWR Morb Mortal Wkly Rep* 1997;46(RR-18):1–42.

Centers for Disease Control and Prevention. Recommendations for preventing transmission of human immunodeficiency virus and hepatitis B virus to patients during exposure-prone invasive procedures. *MMWR Morb Mortal Wkly Rep* 1991;40(RR-8):1–8.

Immunization of Patients with Altered Immunity

Centers for Disease Control and Prevention. Recommendations of the Advisory Committee on Immunization Practices (ACIP): use of vaccines and immune globulins in persons with altered immunocompetence. *MMWR Morb Mortal Wkly Rep* 1993;42(RR-4):1–18.

Vaccine Administration

American Academy of Pediatrics, Committee on Infectious Diseases. Recommended timing of routine immunization for children who have recently received immune globulin preparations. *Pediatrics* 1994;93: 682–685.

Centers for Disease Control. National childhood vaccine injury act: requirements for permanent vaccination records and for reporting of selected events after vaccination. *MMWR Morb Mortal Wkly Rep* 1988;37:197–200.

Centers for Disease Control and Prevention. General recommendations on immunization: recommendations of the Advisory Committee on Immunization Practices (ACIP). *MMWR Morb Mortal Wkly Rep* 1994;43(RR-1):1–38.

Immunization of Persons with Egg Allergies

Greenberg MA, Birx DL. Safe administration of mumps-measles-rubella vaccine in egg-allergic children. *J Pediatr* 1988;113:504–506.

Herman JJ, Radin R, Schneiderman R. Allergic reactions to measles (rubeola) vaccine in patients hypersensitive to egg protein. *J Pediatr* 1983;102:196–199.

Kemp A, Van Asperen P, Mukhi A. Measles immunization in children with clinical reactions to egg proteins. *Am J Dis Child* 1990; 144:33–35.

Lavi S, Zimmerman B, Koren G, et al. Administration of measles, mumps, and rubella virus vaccine (live) to egg-allergic children. *JAMA* 1990;263:269–271.

Adverse Event Reporting

Centers for Disease Control. National childhood vaccine injury act: requirements for permanent vaccination records and for reporting of selected events after vaccination. *MMWR Morb Mortal Wkly Rep* 1988;37:197–200.

Chen RT, Rastogi SC, Mullen JR, et al. The vaccine adverse event reporting system (VAERS). *Vaccine* 1994;12:542–550.

Evans G. National Childhood Vaccine Injury Act: revision of the Vaccine Injury Table. *Pediatrics* 1996;1179–1181.

Public Health Service, Department of Health and Human Services. National Vaccine Injury Compensation Program: revisions and additions to the Vaccine Injury Table—II. Federal Register 1997;62: 7685–7690.

Adverse Events Associated with Vaccines (IOM)

Howson CP, Howe CJ, Fineberg HV, eds. *Adverse effects of pertussis and rubella vaccines.* Washington, DC: National Academy Press, 1991.

Stratton KR, Howe CJ, Johnston RB, eds. *Adverse events associated with childhood vaccines: evidence bearing on causality.* Washington, DC: National Academy Press, 1994.

Prophylaxis

Immune Globulin Products

Immune Globulin (IG)

Centers for Disease Control. Measles prevention: recommendations of the Immunization Practices Advisory Committee (ACIP). *MMWR Morb Mortal Wkly Rep* 1989;39(S-9):1–18.

Centers for Disease Control and Prevention. Prevention of hepatitis A through active or passive immunization: recommendations of the Advisory Committee on Immunization Practices (ACIP). *MMWR Morb Mortal Wkly Rep* 1996:45(RR-15):1–30.

Intravenous Immune Globulin (IVIG)

ASHP Commission on Therapeutics. ASHP therapeutic guidelines for intravenous immune globulin. *Clin Pharmacokinet* 1992;11:117–136.

Ratko TA, Burnett DA, Foulke GE, et al. Recommendations for off-label use of intravenously administered immunoglobulin preparations. *JAMA* 1995;273:1865–1870.

Cytomegalovirus (CMV) IVIG

Centers for Disease Control and Prevention. 1997 USPHS/IDSA guidelines for the prevention of opportunistic infections in persons infected with human immunodeficiency virus. *MMWR Morb Mortal Wkly Rep* 1997;46(RR-12). (Also reprinted in *Clin Infect Dis* 1997;25[suppl 3]:S313–335.)

Rabies Immune Globulin (RIG)

Centers for Disease Control and Prevention. Rabies prevention—United States, 1991: recommendations of the Immunization Practices Advisory Committee (ACIP). *MMWR Morb Mortal Wkly Rep* 1991;40 (RR-3):1–19.

Respiratory Syncytial Virus (RSV) IVIG

American Academy of Pediatrics, Committee on Infectious Diseases, Committee on Fetus and Newborn. Respiratory syncytial virus immune globulin intravenous: indications for use. *Pediatrics* 1997; 99:645–650.

Tetanus Immune Globulin (TIG)

Centers for Disease Control. Diphtheria, tetanus and pertussis. Recommendations for vaccine use and other preventive measures: recommendations of the Advisory Committee on Immunization Practices (ACIP). *MMWR Morb Mortal Wkly Rep* 1991;40(RR-10):1–28.

Varicella-zoster Immune Globulin (VZIG)

American Academy of Pediatrics, Committee on Infectious Diseases. Recommendations for the use of live attenuated varicella vaccine. *Pediatrics* 1995;95:791–796.

Centers for Disease Control and Prevention. Prevention of varicella: recommendations of the Advisory Committee on Immunization Practices (ACIP). *MMWR Morb Mortal Wkly Rep* 1996;45(RR-11):1–36.

Postexposure Prophylaxis

Diphtheria

Centers for Disease Control and Prevention. Diphtheria, tetanus, and pertussis: recommendations for vaccine use and other preventive measures: recommendations of the Immunizations Practices Advisory Committee (ACIP). *MMWR Morb Mortal Wkly Rep* 1991;40(RR-10): 1–28.

Haemophilus influenzae type b

American Academy of Pediatrics, Committee on Infectious Diseases. Revision of recommendation for use of rifampin prophylaxis of contacts of patients with *Haemophilus influenzae* infection. *Pediatrics* 1984;74:301–302.

Hepatitis A

American Academy of Pediatrics, Committee on Infectious Diseases. Prevention of hepatitis A infections: guidelines for use of hepatitis A vaccine and immune globulin. *Pediatrics* 1996;98:1207–1215.

Centers for Disease Control and Prevention. Prevention of hepatitis A through active or passive immunization: recommendations of the Advisory Committee on Immunization Practices (ACIP). *MMWR Morb Mortal Wkly Rep* 1996:45(RR-15):1–30. (Published erratum appears in Centers for Disease Control and Prevention. Erratum: vol. 45, no. RR-15. *MMWR Morb Mortal Wkly Rep* 1997;46:588.)

Hepatitis B

Centers for Disease Control and Prevention. Protection against viral hepatitis: recommendations of the Immunization Practices Advisory Committee (ACIP). *MMWR Morb Mortal Wkly Rep* 1990:39(RR-2): 1–26.

Hepatitis C

Centers for Disease Control and Prevention. Protection against viral hepatitis: recommendations of the Immunization Practices Advisory Committee (ACIP). *MMWR Morb Mortal Wkly Rep* 1990:39(RR-2): 1–26.

Human Immunodeficiency Virus (HIV)

Centers for Disease Control and Prevention. Public Health Service guidelines for the management of health-care worker exposures to HIV and recommendations for postexposure prophylaxis. *MMWR Morb Mortal Wkly Rep* 1998;47(RR-7):1–33.

Influenza Virus

Centers for Disease Control and Prevention. Prevention and control of influenza: recommendations of the Advisory Committee on Immunization Practices (ACIP). *MMWR Morb Mortal Wkly Rep* 1996:45 (RR-5):1–24.

Measles

Centers for Disease Control. Measles prevention: recommendations of the Immunization Practices Advisory Committee (ACIP). *MMWR Morb Mortal Wkly Rep* 1989;39(S-9):1–18.

Meningococcus (*Neisseria meningitidis*)

American Academy of Pediatrics, Committee on Infectious Diseases, and Canadian Paediatric Society, Infectious Diseases and Immunization Committee. Meningococcal disease prevention and control strategies for practice-based physicians. *Pediatrics* 1996;97:404–411.

Centers for Disease Control and Prevention. Control and prevention of meningococcal disease: recommendations of the Advisory Committee on Immunization Practices (ACIP). *MMWR Morb Mortal Wkly Rep* 1997;46(RR-5):1–10.

Centers for Disease Control and Prevention. Control and prevention of serogroup C meningococcal disease: evaluation and management of suspected outbreaks: recommendations of the Advisory Committee on Immunization Practices (ACIP). *MMWR Morb Mortal Wkly Rep* 1997;46(RR-5):13–21.

Plague (*Yersinia pestis*)

Centers for Disease Control and Prevention. Prevention of plague: recommendations of the Advisory Committee on Immunization Practices (ACIP). *MMWR Morb Mortal Wkly Rep* 1996;45(RR-14):1–15.

Rabies

Centers for Disease Control and Prevention. Rabies prevention—United States, 1991: recommendations of the Immunization Practices Advisory Committee (ACIP). *MMWR Morb Mortal Wkly Rep* 1991;40 (RR-3):1–19.

Centers for Disease Control and Prevention. Availability of new rabies vaccine for human use. *MMWR Morb Mortal Wkly Rep* 1998; 47:12, 19.

Tetanus

Centers for Disease Control and Prevention. Diphtheria, tetanus, and pertussis: recommendations for vaccine use and other preventive measures: recommendations of the Immunizations Practices Advisory Committee (ACIP). *MMWR Morb Mortal Wkly Rep* 1991;40(RR-10): 1–28.

Tuberculosis

American Academy of Pediatrics, Committee on Infectious Diseases. Chemotherapy for tuberculosis in infants and children. *Pediatrics* 1992;89:161–165.

American Academy of Pediatrics, Committee on Infectious Diseases. Screening for tuberculosis in infants and children. *Pediatrics* 1994;93: 131–134.

American Academy of Pediatrics, Committee on Infectious Diseases. Update on tuberculosis skin testing of children. *Pediatrics* 1996;97: 282–284.

American Thoracic Society. The tuberculin skin test. *Am Rev Respir Dis* 1981;124:356–363.

American Thoracic Society. Control of tuberculosis. *Am Rev Respir Dis* 1992;146:1623–1633.

American Thoracic Society. Treatment of tuberculosis and tuberculosis infection in adults and children. *Am J Respir Crit Care Med* 1994;149: 1359–1374.

Centers for Disease Control and Prevention. Anergy skin testing and preventive therapy for HIV-infected persons: revised recommendations. *MMWR Morb Mortal Wkly Rep* 1997;46(RR-15):1–10.

Centers for Disease Control and Prevention. Screening for tuberculosis and tuberculosis infection in high-risk populations: recommendations of the Advisory Committee for the Elimination of Tuberculosis. *MMWR Morb Mortal Wkly Rep* 1995;44(RR-11): 19–34.

Varicella-zoster Virus

Centers for Disease Control and Prevention. Prevention of varicella. *MMWR Morb Mortal Wkly Rep* 1996;45(RR-11):1–36.

Prophylaxis for Other Infectious Agents

Follow Infectious Diseases Society of America (IDSA) practice guidelines.

Perinatal Prophylaxis

Ophthalmia neonatorum (gonococcal conjunctivitis)

American Academy of Pediatrics, Committee on Fetus and Newborn, and American College of Obstetricians and Gynecologists, Committee on

Obstetric Practice. *Guidelines for perinatal care,* 4th ed. The Academy, 1997.

Group B *Streptococcus*

American Academy of Pediatrics, Committee on Infectious Diseases and Committee on Fetus and Newborn. Revised guidelines for prevention of early-onset group B streptococcal (GBS) infection. *Pediatrics* 1997;99:489–496.

American College of Obstetricians and Gynecologists. *Group B streptococcal infections in pregnancy.* ACOG technical bulletin no. 170. Washington, DC: American College of Obstetricians and Gynecologists, 1992.

Centers for Disease Control and Prevention. Prevention of perinatal group B streptococcal disease: a public health perspective. *MMWR Morb Mortal Wkly Rep* 1996;45(RR-7):1–24. (Published erratum appears in Centers for Disease Control and Prevention. Erratum: vol. 45, no. RR-7. *MMWR Morb Mortal Wkly Rep* 1996;45:679.)

Hepatitis B

Centers for Disease Control and Prevention. Protection against viral hepatitis: recommendations of the Immunization Practices Advisory Committee (ACIP). *MMWR Morb Mortal Wkly Rep* 1990;39(RR-2): 1–26.

Varicella-zoster Virus (Chickenpox)

Centers for Disease Control and Prevention. Prevention of varicella. *MMWR Morb Mortal Wkly Rep* 1996;45(RR-11):1–36.

HIV-1

Centers for Disease Control and Prevention. Public Health Service task force recommendations for the use of antiretroviral drugs in pregnant women infected with HIV-1 for maternal health and for reducing perinatal HIV-1 transmission in the United States. *MMWR Morb Mortal Wkly Rep* 1998;47(RR-2):1–30.

Perioperative Surgical Prophylaxis

American Academy of Pediatrics, Committee on Infectious Diseases, Committee on Drugs, and Section on Surgery. Antimicrobial prophylaxis in pediatric surgical patients. *Pediatrics* 1984;74: 437–439.

Kaiser AB. Antimicrobial prophylaxis in surgery. *N Engl J Med* 1986; 315:1129–1138.

Antimicrobial prophylaxis in surgery. *Med Lett Drugs Ther* 1997;39: 97–102.

Infective Endocarditis Prophylaxis

Dajani AS, Taubert KA, Wilson W, et al. Prevention of bacterial endocarditis: recommendations by the American Heart Association. *JAMA* 1997;277:1794–1801.

Prophylaxis for Bacterial Infections in Patients with Asplenia

Gaston MH, Verter JI, Woods G, et al. Prophylaxis with oral penicillin in children with sickle cell anemia: a randomized trial. *N Engl J Med* 1986;314:1593–1599.

Falletta JM, Woods GM, Verter JI, et al. Discontinuing penicillin prophylaxis in children with sickle cell anemia. *J Pediatr* 1995;127: 685–690.

Prevention of Rheumatic Fever

Dajani A et al. Treatment of acute streptococcal pharyngitis and prevention of rheumatic fever: a statement for health professionals. Committee on Rheumatic Fever, Endocarditis, and Kawasaki Disease of the Council on Cardiovascular Disease in the Young, the American Heart Association. *Pediatrics* 1995;96:758–764.

Bisno AL, Gerber MA, Gwaltney JM Jr, et al. Diagnosis and management of group A streptococcal pharyngitis: a practice guideline. *Clin Infect Dis* 1997;25:574–583.

Pneumocystis carinii *Prophylaxis*

Centers for Disease Control and Prevention. 1995 Revised guidelines for prophylaxis against *Pneumocystis carinii* pneumonia for children infected with or perinatally exposed to human immunodeficiency virus. *MMWR Morb Mortal Wkly Rep* 1995;44(RR-4).

Prophylaxis for Opportunistic Disease in HIV-Infected Persons

Centers for Disease Control and Prevention. 1995 Revised guidelines for prophylaxis against *Pneumocystis carinii* pneumonia for children infected with or perinatally exposed to human immunodeficiency virus. *MMWR Morb Mortal Wkly Rep* 1995;44(RR-4):1–11.

Centers for Disease Control and Prevention. 1997 USPHS/IDSA guidelines for the prevention of opportunistic infections in persons infected with human immunodeficiency virus. *MMWR Morb Mortal Wkly Rep* 1997;46(RR-12). (Also reprinted in *Clin Infect Dis* 1997;25[Suppl 3]:S313–S335.)

Immunization and Prophylaxis for Travel

Centers for Disease Control. Recommendations for the prevention of malaria among travelers. *MMWR Morb Mortal Wkly Rep* 1991;39(RR-3):1–10.

Centers for Disease Control and Prevention. *Health information for international travel, 1996–97.* U.S. Government publication no. (CDC) 95-8280. Atlanta: Department of Health and Human Services, 1997 (available at www.cdc.gov/travel/yellowbk/).

Isolation Precautions in Hospitals

American Academy of Pediatrics, Committee on Infectious Diseases and Committee on Hospital Care. The revised CDC guidelines for isolation precautions in hospitals: implications for pediatrics. *Pediatrics electronic pages* 1998;101(3):e13.

Centers for Disease Control and Prevention. Guidelines for preventing the transmission of tuberculosis in health-care facilities, 1994. *MMWR Morb Mortal Wkly Rep* 1994;43(RR-13):1–132.

Centers for Disease Control and Prevention. Update: management of patients with suspected viral hemorrhagic fever—United States. *MMWR Morb Mortal Wkly Rep* 1995;44:475–479.

Garner JS, the Hospital Infection Control Practices Advisory Committee. Guideline for isolation precautions in hospitals. *Infect Control Hosp Epidemiol* 1996;17:53–80.

Hospital Infection Control Practices Advisory Committee. Guideline for prevention of nosocomial pneumonia. II. Recommendations for prevention of nosocomial pneumonia. *Am J Infect Control* 1994;22:266–292; and *Infect Control Hosp Epidemiol* 1994;15:604–627.

Tablan OC, Anderson LJ, Arden NH, et al. Guideline for prevention of nosocomial pneumonia. I. Issues on prevention of nosocomial pneumonia—1994. *Am J Infect Control* 1994;22:247–266; and *Infect Control Hosp Epidemiol* 1994;15:587–604.

Vaccination Resources

Updates to This Pocket Guide

www.vaccine.uthscsa.edu

General Vaccine Information

Dennehy PH, Jost EE, Peter G. Active immunizing agents. In Feigin RD, Cherry JD, eds. *Textbook of pediatric infectious diseases*, 4th ed. Philadelphia: Saunders, 1997, pp. 2731–2769.

Fischer GW. Immunotherapy and immunomodulation. In Jenson HB, Baltimore RS, eds. *Pediatric infectious diseases: principles and practice.* Stamford, Conn: Appleton & Lange, 1995, pp. 275–286.

Marchant CD, Kumar ML. Immunizations. In Jenson HB, Baltimore RS, eds. *Pediatric infectious diseases: principles and practice*. Stamford, Conn: Appleton & Lange, 1995, pp. 295–325.
www.pedid.uthscsa.edu

Plotkin SA, Mortimer EA Jr, Orenstein W. *Vaccines,* 3rd ed. Philadelphia: Saunders, 1998.

Stiehm ER. Passive Immunization. In Feigin RD, Cherry JD, eds. *Textbook of pediatric infectious diseases,* 4th ed. Philadelphia: Saunders, 1997, pp. 2769–2802.

American Academy of Pediatrics www.aap.org	800-433-9016
Centers for Disease Control and Prevention (CDC) www.cdc.gov	
National Immunization Program, CDC www.cdc.gov/nip	800-232-2522 800-232-0233 (Spanish)
NIP Education and Training Branch	404-639-8225
Morbidity and Mortality Weekly Report (MMWR) www.cdc.gov/epo/mmwr/mmwr.html	
National Vaccine Injury Compensation Program (VICP) www.hrsa.dhhs.gov/bhpr/vicp/	
World Health Organization www.who.org	

National Vaccine Injury Compensation Program (VICP), Vaccine Adverse Event Reporting System

www.hrsa.dhhs.gov/bhpr/vicp/

Reporting adverse events following vaccination	800-822-7967
Information and general documentation	800-338-2382
Rules of the court; filing a petition	202-219-9657

Vaccine Manufacturers

Aviron (www.aviron.com)	650-919-6500
Chiron (www.chiron.com)	800-244-7668 (800-CHIRON-8)
Connaught	800-822-2463 (800-VACCINE)
Evans Medical/Medeva Pharmaceuticals	800-932-1950
Massachusetts PHBL	617-522-3700, ext. 276
Michigan Biologic Products Institute (BPI)	517-335-8120
Merck (www.merck.com)	800-672-6372
Varicella vaccine	800-982-7482 (800-9-VARIVAX)
North American Vaccine (www.nava.com)	301-419-8400
Organon Teknika	800-323-6442
Parke-Davis	800-223-0432
Pasteur Mérieux Connaught (www.us.pmc-vasc.com)	800-822-2463
SmithKline Beecham (www.sb.com)	
Product information	800-366-8900, ext. 5231
Patient information materials	800-366-8900, ext. 3670
Wyeth-Lederle Vaccines & Pediatrics (www.chp.com)	800-820-2815
Professional Services	800-395-9938
Wyeth-Ayerst Laboratories (FluShield)	800-358-7443

Immune Globulin Manufacturers

Abbott Laboratories	800-323-9100
Alpha Therapeutic	800-421-0008
American Red Cross	800-261-5772
Baxter	800-423-2090
Bayer	800-288-8370
Centeon	800-504-5434
Immuno	810-652-7872
Massachusetts PHBL	617-522-3700, ext. 276
MedImmune	800-949-3789
Michigan BPI	517-335-8119
Miles Laboratories	800-288-8371
New York Blood Center	800-487-8751
Novartis	800-526-0175

Travel Information

Centers for Disease Control and Prevention (CDC)
www.cdc.gov/travel/travel.html

Automated voice information (disease-specific topics)	888-232-3228
Automated Fax information service	888-232-3299 (888-CDC-FAXX)
International travelers' regional recommendations	404-332-4565
Malaria hotline for physicians (8:00 AM–4:30 PM ET)	770-488-7788
After normal business hours	404-639-2888
Immunization hotline for health-care professionals	800-232-7468 (800-CDC-SHOT)
Immunization hotline for consumers	800-232-2522
U.S. State Department travel advisory	202-647-5225

Index

B

C

J

R

S

V

W

Y